LET'S BE REAL ABOUT
REFLUX

Let's Be Real About
REFLUX

Getting To The Heart Of Heartburn

Steven Sandberg-Lewis, ND, DHANP

Portland, Oregon

Cover illustration by Kayle Sandberg-Lewis
Interior illustrations by Kayle Sandberg-Lewis and Asher Sandberg-Lewis
Senior Editor: Kayle Sandberg-Lewis, LMT, MA, BCN Fellow

Book Design and Production:
Fourth Lloyd Productions, LLC, 512 Old Glebe Point Rd., Burgess, VA 22432

For permission to reproduce selections from this book, please write to:
Steven Sandberg-Lewis, ND
P.O. Box 82901
Portland, OR 97282

ISBN: 979-8-218-14784-6
Library of Congress Control Number: 2023902858

Printed in the USA

All disease begins in the gut.

—Aristotle

Table of Contents

FOREWORD

Steven Sandberg-Lewis, ND, is a pathfinder. In this book he dissects all known parameters causing reflux. In fact, his thorough review of the literature and application of his vast naturopathic knowledge expands the field of reflux to hitherto unknown heights.

He starts off with a framework to understand his background as a naturopathic doctor. Ultimately this leads to finding the root cause for each individual who is suffering with "heartburn". All potential aspects of the patient's medical, dietary, behavioral, and pharmacologic history are considered. Exploring all potential causes of reflux will lead to better and more specific treatment.

Students of all types of medicine and doctors in practice can benefit from "digesting" this book from beginning to end. Use of a glossary at the beginning of each chapter allows the lay public to glean all of the lessons in each chapter. The patient then can become an advocate for their health—stop the knee jerk medical approach ("Heartburn? Here is a prescription for a PPI").

There is so much more that Dr. Sandberg-Lewis details in this discourse. Open the book, start reading, and take the deep dive into reflux.

Leonard B. Weinstock, MD

Board certified in internal medicine and gastroenterology

Practicing adult gastroenterology at Specialists in Gastroenterology,
St. Louis, Missouri

Associate Professor of Clinical Medicine,
Washington University School of Medicine, St. Louis, Missouri

Acknowledgements

A giant thank you to Kayle Sandberg-Lewis for all your support, editing, fine illustrations,
and creation of the incredibly important chapter on the alarm system in the brain.
Thanks for being my partner for the last 45 years.

Thanks to Asher for the cartoons and illustrations. They make me smile.
A big thank you to Nancy and Richard Stodart at Fourth Lloyd Productions for their skills,
patience, creativity and sense of humor while turning our manuscript into a fully ready book.
Also thanks to Verla Cowan and Jan Kennedy for pre-reading and suggestions.

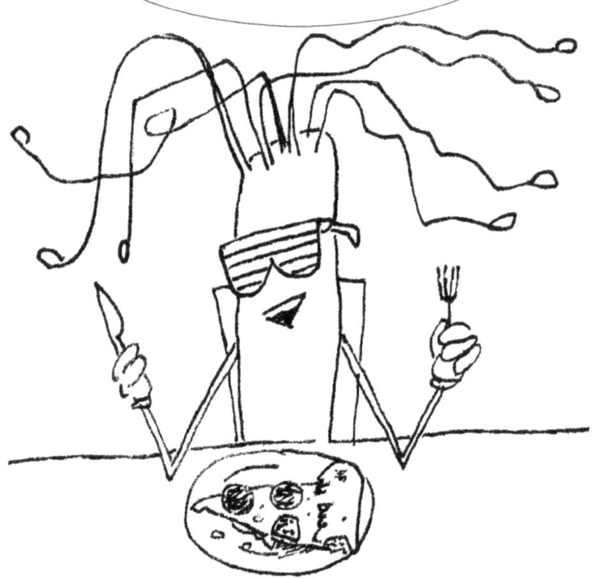
H. pylori may be protective against reflux and its complications.

Introduction

If a hammer is all that you see,
Then a nail every problem will be,
So, reject the poor hammer,
And think in a manner,
That allows things to be seen clearly.

Glossary

hypermobility type Ehlers-Danlos syndrome—a genetic condition affecting protein and resulting in unstable joint structures and lax internal organs

calcium channel blockers—a type of medication used to lower blood pressure by preventing calcium from entering the cells of the heart and arteries

proton pump inhibitors (PPI)—a class of medications that cause a profound and prolonged reduction of stomach acid production

H2 receptor antagonists (H$_2$ blockers)—a class of medications that reduce stomach acid production by blocking the action of histamine on the parietal cells of the stomach.

vagus nerve dysfunction—reduced activity of a key nerve that controls most aspects of digestive function

have practiced **Naturopathic medicine** since the late 1970s and I love my work. I have found my profession gratifying and a real blast as a career. I know of no movie or television series based on the day-to-day practice of a naturopathic physician, let alone a naturopathic gastroenterologist. Shows about doctors are usually about trauma, emergency departments, and life or death stories that keep the viewer on edge as the drama unfolds. While I find my work exciting, neither naturopathic medicine nor GI health and disease has been considered dramatic enough for television, but the truth is diagnosing and treating people with digestive diseases requires real detective work.

Naturopathic Medicine

Naturopathic medicine is grounded in a strong philosophy with basic tenets that naturopathic physicians strive to keep in mind when working with all patients. These include:

First, do no harm.

• This is part of the Hippocratic oath to which all schools of medicine aspire. In Naturopathic medicine, when appropriate, we have many less-toxic options to pursue in order to tailor the treatment to the individual needs of the patient

Prevention.

• An ounce of this is worth a pound of cure

Holism—treat the whole patient

• The body is more than the sum of its parts. Systems of the body interact from the subcellular level up to the whole. Physical, mental, emotional and spiritual components are all important factors.

Doctor as teacher.

• The word doctor comes from the Latin verb "**docere**," meaning to teach

• If physicians share important concepts of health and disease, the process becomes more internally guided for the patient. This makes it possible for the doctor and patient to work together to get a better outcome.

The healing power of nature.

• Organisms have an energy that directs maintenance, repair and healing

• Symptoms are often the body's best attempt at protecting and healing itself

Treat the cause whenever possible.

• Don't just focus on symptoms

Much has changed in medicine over the last four decades, but these principles have proved enduring and have provided an overarching framework that has guided me as I have evolved as a physician. In writing this book, two of the above tenets are of particular importance to me.

Treat the Cause

A frequent complaint from patients is that their previous doctors simply prescribed symptom suppressive treatments. I can't speak for other physicians, but there is a tendency in Western medicine

Treating the cause, whenever possible, is a strong focus for me and other naturopathic physicians.

(biomedicine) to rely on brief primary care visits with the expectation that a prescription will be written to address one or more symptoms at the conclusion of most appointments. That model doesn't allow the time necessary to thoroughly investigate the cause(s) of the complaints.

Treating the cause, whenever possible, is a strong focus for me and other naturopathic physicians. For example, there are risk factors that may underly digestive disorders, while other risk factors can make existing digestive diseases more complex. Knowing to check for these factors gives me a deeper understanding of a patient's situation and a clearer path to helping.

A partial list of risk factors I investigate with each new patient includes the following:

In cases that have resisted successful treatment, there are often multiple causes and underlying factors complicating the picture.

A careful analysis can allow rational use of interventions that lead to effective results and avoid the triggering of new diseases.

Bold words in the text are defined in the glossary.

- hypermobility syndromes such as **hypermobility type Ehlers-Danlos syndrome**
- history of medication use including those that alter the microbiome (steroids, antibiotics—especially extended continuous use for acne or recurrent urinary tract infection)
- history of use of drugs that slow down the gut (narcotics, **calcium channel blockers**, antidiarrheals and antispasmodics other than peppermint oil)
- altered anatomy (congenital, acquired or surgical changes in the structures of the gut)
- history of use of drugs that alter digestive secretions (**proton pump inhibitors, H2 receptor antagonists**)
- GI valve/sphincter dysfunction (lower esophageal, pyloric, ileocecal, anal)
- thyroid or adrenal gland imbalances
- history of perforated abdominal or pelvic organs or surgeries that may stimulate adhesion formation
- internal bleeding including endometriosis
- **vagus nerve dysfunction**
- immune system suppression (from immune suppressive medication or immune system disease)
- histamine sensitivity or mast cell activation syndrome

- inflammation or thickening of the intestines (ie. scleroderma, Crohn's disease)

- blood sugar and insulin dysregulation (insulin resistance, hypoglycemia, prediabetes or diabetes)

- birth mode (cesarean, forceps extraction) and early feeding details (lack of breast feeding, use of formula, early introduction of solid foods)

- history of food poisoning, traveler's diarrhea or gastroenteritis

- mold illness or certain tickborne infections

- overtraining exercise patterns with excessively high pulse rate

- digestive pH abnormalities or enzyme deficiencies

- history of traumatic brain injury

In cases that have resisted successful treatment there are often multiple causes and underlying factors complicating the picture. A careful analysis can allow rational use of interventions that lead to effective results and avoid the triggering of new diseases.

Doctor as Teacher

Early in my career, I held lectures and workshops for my patients to help them gain self-care tools. I continue to consider every patient contact an educational opportunity. After about ten years in practice, I started teaching at naturopathic colleges. In 2009 I published the first edition of my textbook *Functional Gastroenterology—Assessing and Addressing the Causes of Functional Gastrointestinal Disorders*. It was my best effort at focusing on health and wellness with little emphasis on specific diseases. By that time, I had been teaching pathology for seventeen years and wanted to shift gears to explain my approach to optimizing the health of the GI tract rather than describing GI diseases. Because the textbook has been well received, I have been invited to teach at a variety of national and international conferences.

Although *Let's Be Real About Reflux: Getting to the Heart of Heartburn* is not a textbook, I present a full explanation of heartburn, from causes to treatments. It is my hope that patients and physicians alike will find it informative.

Part of the confusion regarding reflux is that the symptom of heartburn and other reflux symptoms can be caused by many things, only one of them being acid reflux.

This book is meant to provide a real understanding of reflux and legitimate options for treatment.

Heartburn is an extremely common issue. It is a key symptom for a group of GI diseases under the umbrella term "gastroesophageal reflux". I named this book *Let's Be Real About Reflux* because the subject is ridiculously simplified in most of the current literature as well as in the minds of many physicians and patients. The simplification often leads to seeing all heartburn as reflux. That viewpoint leads to a prescription for a proton pump inhibitor without any attempt to find or address the cause(s) of the heartburn. Often heartburn is assumed to be a symptom of too much acid, but heartburn is just a symptom. It may be caused by a variety of issues.

Part of the confusion regarding reflux is that the symptom of heartburn and other reflux symptoms can be caused by many things, only one of them being acid reflux. If the "diagnosis" of GERD is made with a hunch and a PPI challenge or just a questionnaire, the accuracy is wrong up to 37% of the time. If a gastroenterologist rather than a family practice physician makes the diagnosis, the accuracy is, on average, improved by only 7%. Let's be real about reflux and get to the heart of heartburn.

As you read this book, an important concept to understand is the pH scale as shown below. pH refers to power or potential of hydrogen. The concentration of the hydrogen ion in a solution determines the pH.

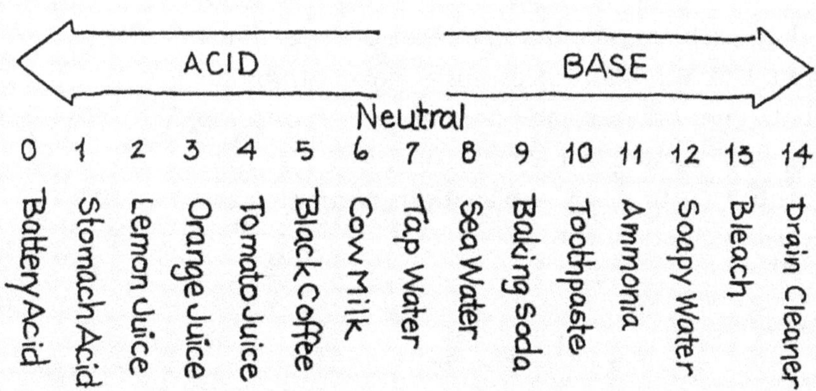

The pH scale ranges from 0-14. For example, water is typically found to have a pH of 7; human blood about 7.4. Up to 6.9 is the acid range with acidity increasing as the numbers get lower. Typical healthy acid pH of the stomach is under 2.0, Hypochlorhydria is generally a pH greater than 3.0. Bacterial overgrowth in the stomach occurs when the pH is greater than 3.8. Alkaline (also called basic) pH ranges from 7.1-14.0 with alkalinity increasing as the numbers increase. Baking soda (sodium bicarbonate) solutions are about pH 9.0. The goal of proton pump inhibitors is to raise the pH from below 2.0 to above 6.0 for at least 19 hours per day—therefore these medications are designed to induce significant hypochlorhydria.

HOW IS pH MEASURED?

You may remember from your science classes using pH paper, usually small strips, to test the acid/base level of a substance. pH paper is chemically treated to reveal through color changes whether a substance is acid (represented by red tones) or alkaline (represented by shades of blue). The deeper the color, the stronger the response. These strips can be used to measure the pH of saliva or vaginal secretions and are a component of urine "dipsticks" which are used to check urine pH, in addition to concentration, protein, sugar, bilirubin, ketones and markers of infection.

There are also more sophisticated instruments that measure pH. They are used when gastroenterologists test the pH of the upper digestive tract. Chapter four covers the various tests used.

THE LAYOUT OF THE BOOK

For you to get the most from this book, each chapter begins with its own glossary of terms and "key questions" to help you focus. I've tried to build on each chapter, but if you prefer to read just what interests you, I have reinforced essential details throughout. Drawings, both light-hearted and informative, are scattered throughout along with some groan-worthy limericks. It is my sincere desire you benefit from my explanations and enjoy the process.

ONE

HOW THE UPPER DIGESTIVE SYSTEM SHOULD WORK: ANATOMY AND PHYSIOLOGY

The mouth starts digestion by chewing.
The teeth grind the food and, ungluing,
It adds amylase
From inside your face—
Not chewing may be your undoing.

GLOSSARY

ampulla of Vater—a nipple-like protrusion in the duodenum out of which pancreatic and bile fluids flow from the common bile duct into the intestine

angle of His—the angle formed where the stomach meets the esophagus. This shape reinforces the integrity of the LES and allows the stomach to fit against the underside of the diaphragm

antibody—a protein produced by the body's immune system which detects harmful organisms or substances and binds to them

antrum—the lowest portion of the stomach which leads to the pyloric valve

body of stomach— the largest and middle portion of the stomach

bolus—a rounded mass of chewed food mixed with saliva

brush border—the mucus membrane lining the small intestine with multiple tiny finger-like projections

cardiac notch—another name for the angle of His

chief cells—stomach cells that produce the enzyme pepsin

defensins—a group of immune system proteins that kill microorganisms

fundus—the top of the stomach; area above the angle of His

gastric acid—hydrochloric acid produced in the parietal cells of the stomach

gastrin—a hormone produced in the antrum of the stomach, gastrin has the ability to stimulate gastric acid production

histamine—a proinflammatory substance produced by certain white blood cells and gut bacteria as well as cells in the body of the stomach

intrinsic factor—a substance produced in the stomach which is essential for absorption of vitamin B12

lactoferrin—an iron binding protein in the digestive secretions that controls the growth of bacteria and fungi

lower esophageal sphincter (LES)—the valve at the bottom of the esophagus that prevents reflux of stomach contents

lysozyme—an enzyme in digestive secretions that kills bacteria

masticated—chewed

pepsin—a stomach enzyme that starts the digestion of protein

peristalsis—coordinated muscle contractions that move food through the digestive tract

peristaltic—referring to peristalsis

physiological reflux—minimal amounts of reverse flow in the digestive tract that do not cause symptoms or disease

primary esophageal contractions—the esophageal peristaltic wave triggered by swallowing

pylorus or pyloric sphincter—the valve between the stomach and duodenum

secondary esophageal contractions—a reflex peristaltic wave triggered when swallowed material does not completely clear the esophagus

secretory IgA—an antibody secreted into GI fluids that binds and inactivates certain microorganisms and food proteins

stratified squamous—layers of flat cells that form the inner lining of the esophagus

upper esophageal sphincter—a thickened area of muscle in the upper esophagus

KEY QUESTIONS

What are the basic structures and functions of the upper digestive tract?

How and why does pH vary throughout the digestive tract?

UNDERSTANDING THE UPPER GASTROINTESTINAL (GI) TRACT

To understand how reflux occurs, it is important to become familiar with the GI tract and how it is supposed to function. Reviewing the anatomy of the tract will help to understand how things can go wrong. The drawing shown on the right is a representation of the entire digestive tract as if it were in a straight line.

THE MOUTH

Digestion starts in the mouth. While mechanically breaking down food by chewing is a vital part of the picture, the chemical process starts here too.

Saliva is crucial for digestion and for preventing irritation from reflux. Each day the salivary glands (parotid, submandibular, sublingual, and minor salivary) produce over a liter of saliva, which is swallowed throughout the day. Healthy saliva is slightly alkaline (pH 7.5). It bathes the esophagus which helps to neutralize any acid reflux that does occur. Saliva contains amylase, an enzyme that starts the digestion of carbohydrates into sugars.

Saliva also contains **defensins**, **secretory IgA** and other antibodies, **lysozyme** and **lactoferrin**—all of which have a protective role for the lining of the esophagus, the tube that transports the food to the stomach. Once the food is chewed and saturated with saliva, it is

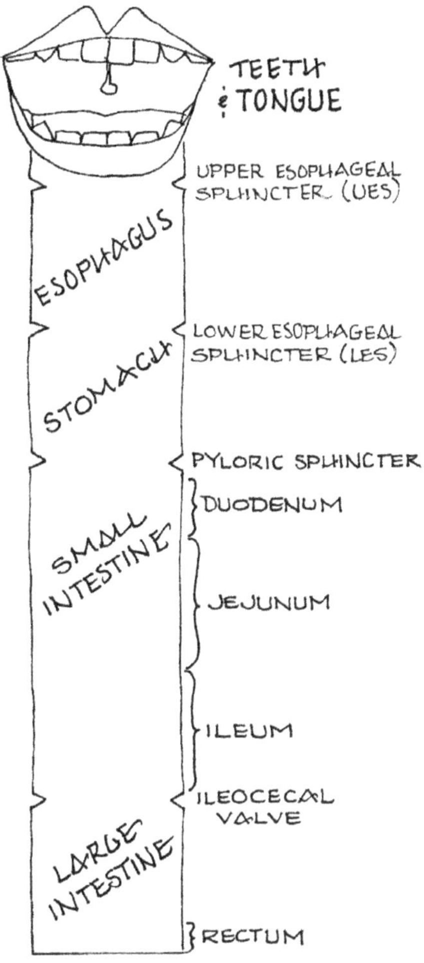

Fig. 1.1. Representation of the entire digestive tract..

Saliva is crucial for digestion and for preventing irritation from reflux.

The salivary glands produce over a liter of saliva per day.

swallowed, a voluntary act, meaning the muscles used to swallow are controlled by intention. The **masticated** mass is called a **bolus** and starts its journey from the pharynx down the esophagus. The first two-thirds of the esophagus respond to the will to swallow, but the lowest third contains only involuntary muscle.

When the bolus enters the lower third of the esophagus, the autonomic nervous system takes over, controlling the peristaltic muscle contractions for you. This involuntary musculature (known as smooth muscle) persists throughout the rest of the digestive tract except for conscious control over the anal sphincter at the very end. Along the esophagus—a tube about ¾ of an inch (2 centimeters) in diameter and 11–13 inches (28–33 centimeters) in length—the elegant rippling of the muscles moves the bolus toward the stomach. This coordinated movement is called **peristalsis**. The first phase of peristalsis is called **primary esophageal contractions.** If the bolus doesn't make it all the way to the stomach, **secondary esophageal contractions** take over and complete the process. Both primary and secondary contractions are normal processes in the esophagus.

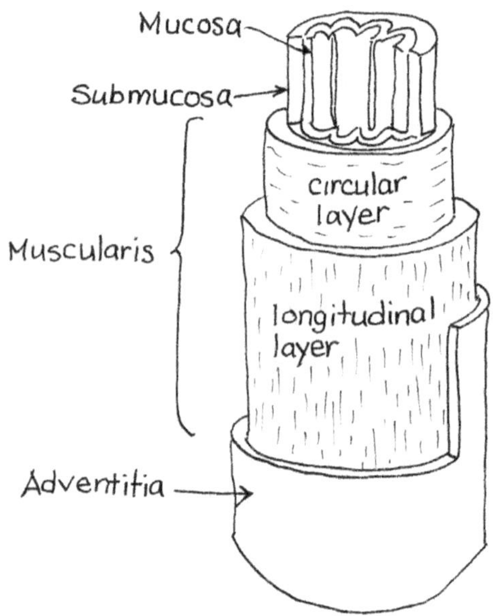

Fig. 1.2. Layers of the esophageal wall.

From the mouth to the anus, the digestive tract is one continuous, multilayered tube. The innermost layer of the tube is called the mucosa or mucus membrane.

Microscopically, the cells lining the esophageal mucosa are called **stratified squamous** and are made up of multiple layers of flattened cells, much like the skin on the back of the hand. They protect the nerves deeper in the esophagus from the food, fluid and microorganisms passing by. Below the stratified squamous layer is the submucosa which contains blood vessels and mucus-producing cells that lubricate and protect the mucosal surface. Deeper than the submucosa is a layer of muscles. These muscles create the **peristaltic** waves that move food down the esophagus. Lastly there is an outer wrapping called adventitia which encloses the entire esophagus, providing structural support.

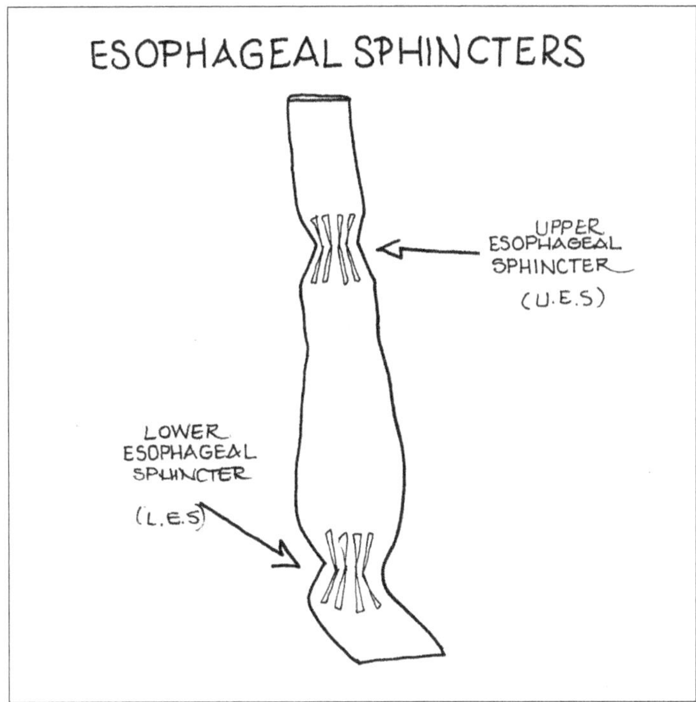

Fig. 1.3. Illustration of the esophageal sphincters.

The LES keeps stomach contents from returning to the esophagus, preventing excessive reflux.

The **upper esophageal sphincter** (UES) is a thickened area of muscle in the upper esophagus that acts like a purse string, cinching the tube to keep swallowed air from getting into the stomach. Excessive air in the stomach can cause uncomfortable pressure, bloating, and repeated burping.

At the junction of the esophagus and stomach, there is another cinch in the muscle called the lower esophageal sphincter (LES). It keeps stomach contents from returning to the esophagus, preventing excessive reflux. A small amount of food or liquid normally comes back through the LES. This is physiological reflux because it does not cause symptoms and the lining of the esophagus is not damaged by its presence. The mucosal surface is protected by saliva, the cells lining the esophagus, and the mucus and bicarbonate produced by the glands in the submucosa. Adequate blood flow in the submucosa helps carry away any acid that may get through this mucosal barrier (Kaunitz JD, 2005).

A higher volume or frequency of return of stomach contents may overpower these protective mechanisms causing the physiological reflux to become pathological. When that occurs, GER becomes GERD, the D denoting disease.

THE STOMACH

The stomach is an elegant bag composed of three layers of muscle with a mucus membrane inner lining. It holds an average of 1.5 liters of food or fluid. After swallowing, the bolus travels down the esophagus and enters the stomach. In the stomach, food is mixed with **gastric acid*** and the enzyme **pepsin**. These substances start the process of digesting protein and prepare minerals for absorption further down the digestive system.

A third substance produced by the stomach lining is **intrinsic factor**, which is part of the complex process needed to absorb vitamin B12.

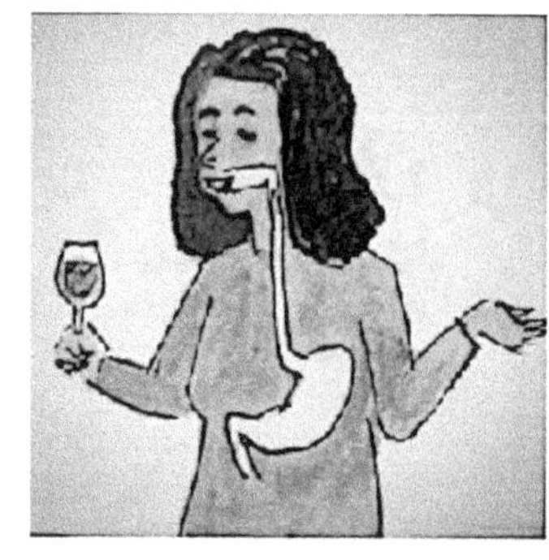

Fig. 1.4.
Illustration of mouth to stomach.

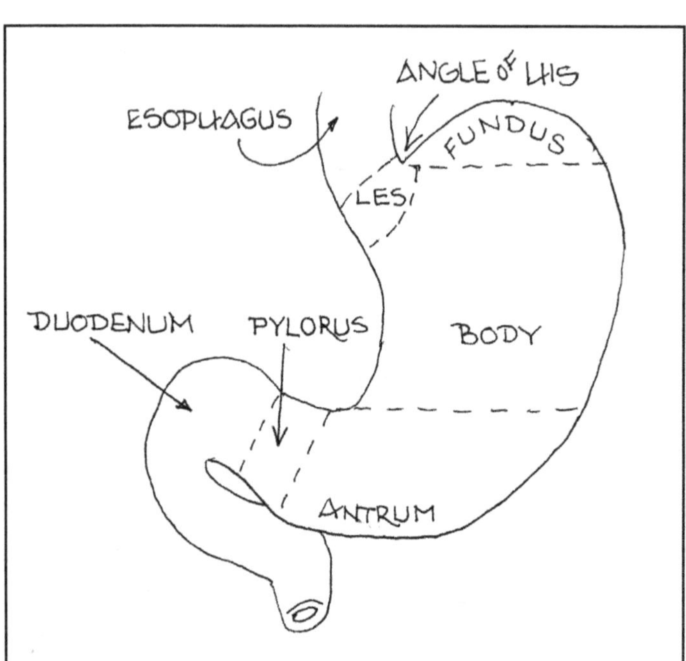

Fig. 1.5. Stomach anatomy.

A properly functioning stomach produces strong acid and enzymes capable of digesting the stomach lining itself, as happens in erosions or ulcers.

As illustrated, the stomach is divided into three regions based on function and types of cells that comprise each area. From the top down are the fundus, body and antrum. The **fundus** is especially important because of the shape of the angle where the stomach meets the esophagus. Called the **cardiac notch** or **angle of His**, it reinforces the integrity of the LES. The angle creates a perfect shape for the fundus of the stomach to fit against the underside of the left dome of the diaphragm. This anatomical feature limits reflux from the stomach into the esophagus.

---

*Hydrochloric acid will be discussed in more detail in chapters five and fourteen.

To protect against the erosive effects of acid and pepsin, the stomach lining has an especially dense extra layer of mucus that is not present in the esophagus or small intestine.

Further down is the body of the stomach where the bolus is mixed with acid and enzymes. This muscular mixing process resembles a shirt sleeve repeatedly being turned inside out and then right side out. The mucus membrane in this area contains **chief cells** which make **pepsin**, and **parietal cells** which make hydrochloric acid as well as intrinsic factor.

The lowest area of the stomach is the **antrum** which is a narrowed area containing special cells that produce **gastrin**, a hormone that stimulates the parietal cells to create more acid. At the very end of the antrum, is the **pyloric sphincter**, another cinch in the muscle. Just as the **lower esophageal sphincter** (LES) at the top of the stomach separates the esophagus from the stomach, the pyloric sphincter separates the stomach from the duodenum.

A properly functioning stomach produces strong acid and enzymes capable of digesting the stomach lining itself, as happens in erosions or ulcers. To protect against this, two special layers of mucus separate the stomach contents from the mucus membrane. In the esophagus, there are not two special layers of mucus, but a mucus/bicarbonate mixture is produced in the submucosa. Blood flowing through the submucosal capillaries may carry away some acid that makes it through these protective layers.

THE DUODENUM

Just beyond the pylorus is the duodenum—the first part of the small intestine.

The duodenum is 10-15 inches long and shaped like the letter "C". In its upper portions, a nipple-like protrusion called the **ampula of Vater** transports pancreatic and bile fluids into the intestine. Pancreatic fluid contains digestive enzymes that break down proteins, fats, and carbohydrates. Additionally, bicarbonate serves to neutralize gastric acid as it enters the duodenum. This creates a slightly alkaline environment which is necessary to activate the pancreatic enzymes. The surface of the mucus membrane lining the small intestine is often referred to as the **brush border** due to its multiple tiny finger-like projections. The brush border produces its own enzymes which finish the digestion of carbohydrates and break down **histamine**.

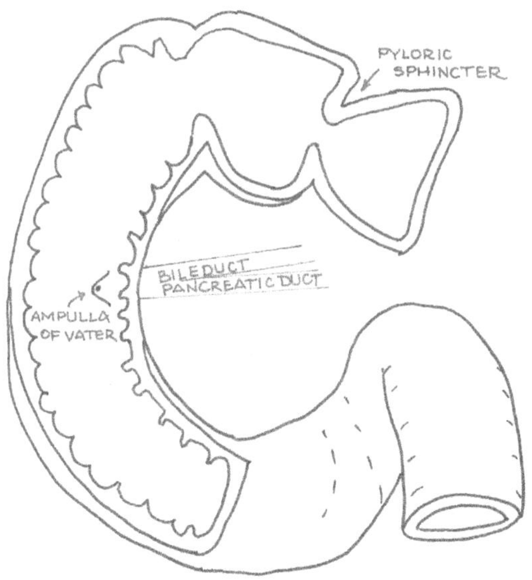

Fig. 1.6. The duodenum.

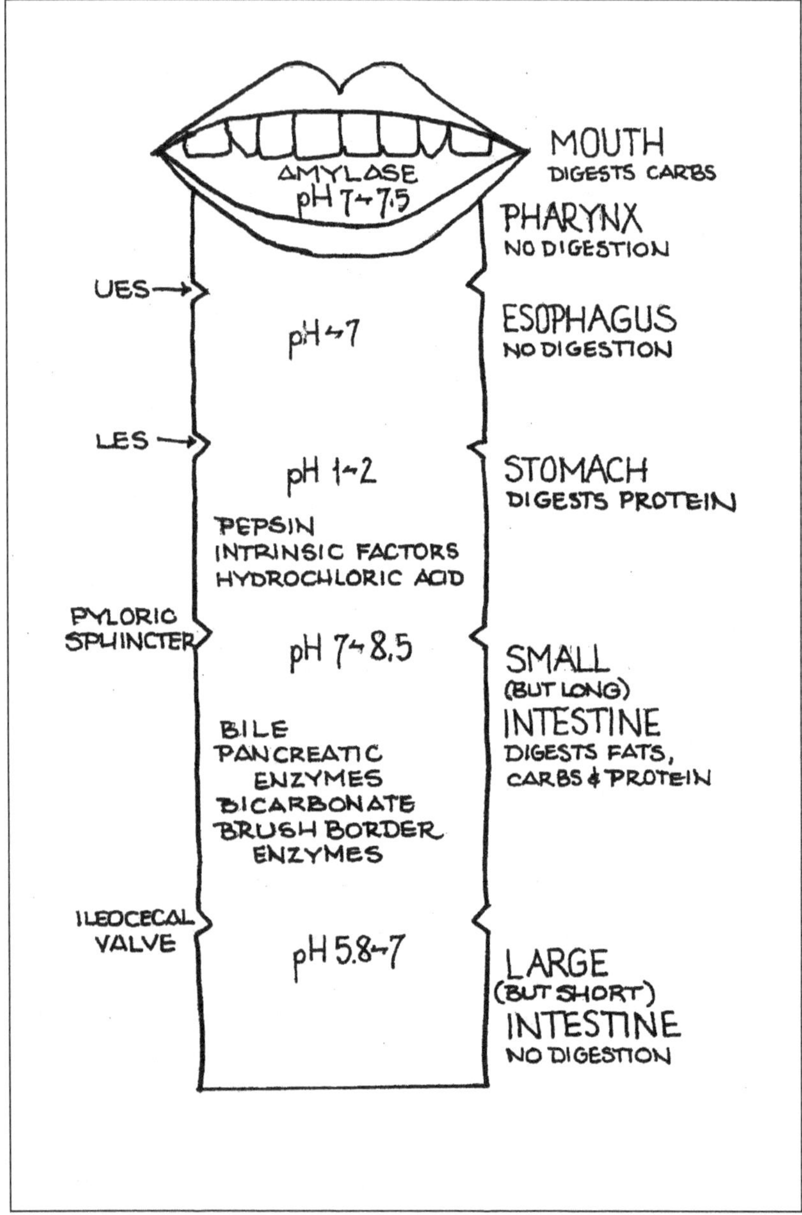

Fig. 1.7. Location of digestive enzymes, acid, bicabonate, and bile in the GI tract.

There are dramatic fluctuations in pH as portions of the GI tract switch from alkaline to acid.

Many patients have told me they are "too acidic" or "too alkaline", but these terms are generally meaningless when referring to the entire tract.

TWO

REFLUX IS NOT SYNONYMOUS WITH HEARTBURN

When people's guts do churn,
A symptom of much, you'll soon learn,
They may call it "GERD",
A diagnostic word.
It's more apt to just say "heartburn".

GLOSSARY

aspiration pneumonia is a lung infection due to inhaling stomach fluid or other substances into the lungs

Barrett's esophagus—cellular changes in the esophagus caused by chronic GERD

biopsy—a microscopic examination of tissue removed from a living body to discover the presence, cause, or extent of a disease.

bicarbonate—a chemical substance produced in various tissues including the saliva and pancreatic fluid. It buffers acids to create a more neutral pH

bile reflux—the backing up of bile from the small intestine into the stomach

cholecystectomy—surgical removal of the gallbladder

chyme—a mixture of gastric fluids and partially digested food

dysphagia—difficulty with the process of swallowing

dysplasia—the presence of cells of an abnormal type within a tissue, which may signify a stage preceding the development of cancer.

endoscopy—the use of a flexible scope to examine the internal lining of organs.

esophagitis—inflammation of the esophagus, especially the mucosa or innermost lining

erosive esophagitis—esophageal inflammation that causes a shallow loss of surface tissue due to chronic GERD

esophageal ulcer—a deeper loss of esophageal surface tissue

gastric compliance or receptive relaxation—the ability of the stomach to fill and stretch to accommodate incoming solid food and liquids.

gastroenterology—the healthcare specialty focusing on diseases of the digestive tract

impaction—the process of food getting stuck in the esophagus

intrathoracic pressure—the pressure within the chest

laryngopharyngeal reflux—a type of reflux sometimes referred to as "**silent reflux**" because there may not be heartburn or typical reflux symptoms. Instead, the symptoms involve the throat or voice.

lingual tonsils—a group of small tonsils on the base of the tongue

metaplasia—transformation of cells from one fully developed form to another. In Barrett's esophagus the metaplasia is transformation from esophageal lining cells to those that normally line the small intestine

non-erosive reflux disease (NERD)—a normal appearance of the esophagus in spite of significant reflux

pH/impedance reflux monitoring—a procedure that measures the amount of reflux (both acidic and non-acidic) in the esophagus during a 24-hour period. A more detailed explanation is found in chapter four.

physiological reflux—the normal minimal backflow of stomach contents into the lower esophagus which does not lead to any esophageal problems

receptive relaxation—decreased stomach muscle tone that allows food to enter and fill the stomach

reflux esophagitis—esophageal inflammation caused by GERD

reflux—the flow of a fluid through a vessel or valve in the body in a direction opposite to normal. In the digestive tract reflux can occur:

> between the stomach and esophagus which is referred to as gastroesophageal reflux; between the small intestine and the stomach, called either bile reflux or duodenal gastric reflux; between the large intestine (cecum) and ileum of the small intestine known as either cecoileal reflux or open ileocecal valve syndrome.

Rome criteria—created by an international group of clinicians, these guidelines standardize diagnosis of functional digestive disorders such as irritable bowel syndrome

silent reflux—gastroesophageal reflux in which typical symptoms such as heartburn are not present

upper endoscopy—a common term for esophagogastroduodenoscopy (EGD) which is a scope that is put into the mouth and extended down to allow examination of the esophagus, stomach, and duodenum.

KEY QUESTIONS

What are the common symptoms of GERD?

What are the various types of reflux?

What are the causes of heartburn besides reflux?

Is heartburn the same thing as GERD?

Some of the more common symptoms of gastroesophageal reflux are: heartburn, regurgitation, chronic cough, sore throat, hoarseness, and chronic throat clearing.

HEARTBURN

People describe heartburn in different ways—burning, sharp, pressing; simply uncomfortable or downright painful. It occurs in the chest, most commonly near the breastbone. *Persistent heartburn is not normal.* It is a symptom that something is wrong. It may be minimal or so severe that it needs to be differentiated from angina or a heart attack. The symptom of heartburn can also occur without abnormal reflux of stomach contents.

Many people are mistakenly diagnosed with gastroesophageal reflux disease (GERD) when their heartburn is a symptom of something else. Reflux is a physiological process in which the contents (liquid, solid, or aerosolized liquid) move up from the stomach into the esophagus or higher.

Gastroesophageal reflux (GER) is the backing up of some of the stomach contents into the esophagus.

Physiological gastroesophageal reflux is a normal phenomenon which happens several times after each meal.

This normal reflux should cause no heartburn or other symptoms because it is buffered by alkaline saliva and esophageal mucus.

Heartburn occurs at least once a week in about 30% of North Americans. (Richter JE, 2018 and Delshad SD, 2020). It is more common in non-Hispanic whites, females, people ages 30-60 years, married and earning $50,000-$100,000 compared to those making more or less than that income bracket (I have no idea why this income bracket has more GERD).

The flow of material through the gastrointestinal tract is described as a north to south process. It takes swallowed food, called a bolus, and liquids about ten seconds to reach the stomach. As the bolus moves through the esophagus it triggers **receptive relaxation** of the upper stomach muscles which increases the volume capacity for incoming food. Within the stomach the food is manipulated by mixing waves that move it forward to the antrum of the stomach, followed by retropulsion which pushes the material back upward to the body of the stomach. As in a clothes washer, the muscles in the wall of the stomach agitate the food, mixing it with acid and pepsin and turning it into **chyme**. Over a four-to-five-hour period, the chyme gradually leaves the stomach and is squirted into the duodenum.

As the chyme moves along the small intestine it is agitated back and forth in a process called segmentation contraction. This mixes the chyme with **bicarbonate** and enzymes. The bulk of the nutrients in the chyme are absorbed from the small intestine into the blood.

The chyme is gradually transforming into stool and enters the large intestine where the back-and-forth mixing continues in sections called haustra. Water and minerals are absorbed into the blood. Finally, indigestible fiber, sloughed off cells of the digestive lining, as well as dead and living bacteria come out in the stool.

Periodically, while the stomach is empty, cleansing waves known as the **migrating motor complex** flush microorganisms and any undigested food though the 18-20 feet of small intestine.

Gastroesophageal Reflux (GER)

Gastroesophageal reflux (GER) is the backing up of some of the stomach contents into the esophagus. Physiological gastroesophageal reflux is a *normal* phenomenon which happens several times after each meal. This normal reflux should cause no heartburn or other symptoms because it is buffered by alkaline saliva and esophageal mucus. Any fluid is moved back down into the stomach by secondary esophageal contractions.

Sometimes the word *reflex* is confused with the word *reflux*. Reflex is an unrelated word defined as an involuntary movement in response to a stimulus. An example of this is blinking when something flies toward one's eye.

Gastroesophageal Reflux Disease (GERD)

Gastroesophageal reflux disease (GERD) is reflux that leads to symptoms, esophageal tissue injury, or both.

Many people use the terms reflux and GERD interchangeably. In general parlance, reflux refers to gastroesophageal reflux, but there are other types of reflux in the digestive tract. Bile reflux is described in chapter seventeen.

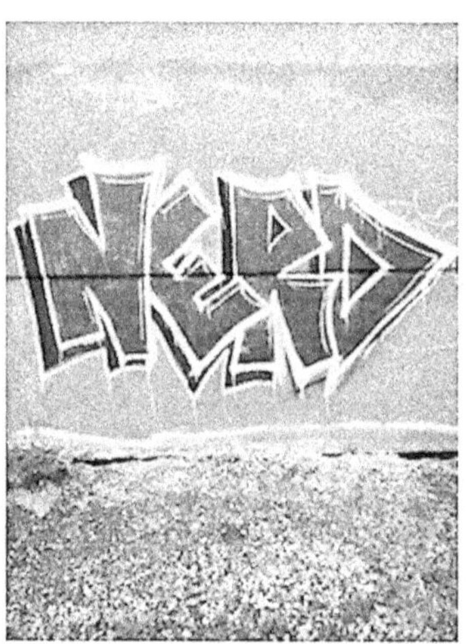

Most patients with GERD show no abnormalities of the esophagus when examined by a gastroenterologist using upper **endoscopy**. This condition is called **non-erosive reflux disease** (NERD). With NERD, people have heartburn and true reflux proven by a test called pH impedance monitoring, but they have no esophageal disease visible either via endoscopy or biopsy. This normal appearance may be attributable to the body's protective mechanisms that prevent damage to the mucus membrane of the esophagus.

Most patients with significant reflux have no visible changes or microscopic damage to the esophagus. This normal appearance is called NERD.

Higher levels of the hormone melatonin may protect the lower esophagus from erosion.

Although only a minority of patients with GERD have measurable disease in the lower esophagus, it is important to keep this population in mind. These changes can range from minimal to severe. The mildest changes in the lower esophagus are redness of the tissue lining which is called **esophageal erythema**. This is the result of increased blood in the capillaries of the gastric lining.

Increased severity involves a superficial wearing away of the esophageal lining, called **erosive esophagitis** or **reflux esophagitis**. Grade A esophagitis is the mildest form of reflux esophagitis and grade D is the most extensive. Even deeper wearing away of the esophageal lining is called an **esophageal ulcer** which is less common.

Another response to chronic reflux is a change in the type of cells lining the esophagus which is called **metaplasia**. Metaplasia in the esophagus is referred to as **Barrett's esophagus** and is the esophageal lining's best attempt to protect itself against long term exposure to stomach contents. Over a longer period, such as many years, a tiny fraction of Barrett's cases can progress to **dysplasia,** a precancerous change, or, even further, to esophageal cancer. The good news is that these more severe complications of GERD are quite rare (0.4-0.5% per year) and effective early treatment often prevents dysplasia and cancer.

Bile Reflux

Bile reflux occurs when the pyloric valve fails to keep bile from backing up into the stomach. This type of reflux is abnormal, and usually starts after **cholecystectomy**. Bile reflux often causes pain, reduced appetite and nausea, with or without vomiting. The bile may continue upward from the stomach and become an additional component of gastroesophageal reflux. See chapter seventeen for a full discussion of bile reflux.

Laryngopharyngeal Reflux (LPR)

A common variation of GERD is laryngopharyngeal reflux (LPR). This is sometimes referred to as **"silent reflux"** because there may not be heartburn or typical reflux symptoms. Instead, the symptoms involve the throat or voice. The symptoms include some combination of

- chronic throat clearing
- cough
- sore throat or spasms
- feeling of suffocation
- bad breath
- sensation of a lump in the throat
- **aspiration pneumonia**
- **dysphagia**
- hoarseness and other changes in the voice
- enlarged **lingual tonsils**

CT scans of adults with laryngopharyngeal reflux (LPR) have

revealed that the average lingual tonsil size was three-fold or greater than people without LPR (Friedman M, 2010). LPR is sometimes diagnosed by an ear, nose and throat specialist (otolaryngologist) rather than a gastroenterologist.

Symptoms and Conditions Mistaken for GERD

There are several syndromes and diseases that are mistaken for reflux. This section explains esophageal conditions that are NOT GERD.

Functional Heartburn

Those with functional heartburn show no evidence of reflux with advanced testing, and no pathological esophageal changes visible through endoscopy or biopsy. Unlike those with reflux hypersensitivity, there is no correlation between their symptoms and physiological reflux. Why these people experience heartburn is not well understood.

Reflux Hypersensitivity

Heartburn in patients who have only **physiological reflux** is called **reflux hypersensitivity**. Even though there is evidence of only physiological reflux, (no pathological reflux), the patient clearly has reflux symptoms in response to the normal presence of back-flow from the stomach.

Physiological reflux alone can cause heartburn in those with reflux hypersensitivity.

TABLE 2.1. How pH Impedance Testing Clarifies GERD Diagnosis		
Heartburn Normal endoscopy and biopsy ▼ GERD is not yet proven ▼ Esophageal pH impedance test is performed clarifying the following causes of heartburn		
Functional Heartburn	**Reflux Hypersensitivity**	**GERD**
Normal reflux of fluid in the esopha-gus and heartburn symptoms **do not** correlate with any reflux of fluid	Normal reflux of fluid in the esophagus but heartburn symptoms **do** correlate with reflux of fluid	Abnormal reflux of fluid in the esophagus and heartburn symptoms **may or may not** correlate with the reflux of fluid

RUMINATION SYNDROME

Rumination syndrome is a rare condition in which food from a previous meal suddenly comes up into the mouth. It is sometimes misdiagnosed as vomiting, although the typical events associated with true vomiting are not present. There is no nausea or retching. Often the food does not taste acidic. It simply rises into the mouth the way a ruminant animal such as a cow would rechew and reprocess food. Rumination syndrome is neither GERD nor vomiting and, according to the **Rome diagnostic criteria**, is considered one of the functional gastrointestinal disorders. It is most successfully treated with diaphragmatic breathing exercises and biofeedback training to normalize the autonomic nervous system.

GLOBUS SENSATION

A persistent or intermittent non-painful sensation, like a lump or a foreign body in the throat, that has been present for at least six months is called globus sensation or phenomenon. According to the Rome diagnostic criteria, there is no evidence that either GERD or other disease process is causing the symptoms. It may be related to anxiety which causes altered salivary flow and therefore less lubrication of the throat.

FUNCTIONAL CHEST PAIN

Functional chest pain is defined by the Rome criteria as chest pain or discomfort behind the breastbone without symptoms of heartburn or difficulty swallowing. As is the case with functional heartburn, there is also no evidence of GERD or other disease process.

EOSINOPHILIC ESOPHAGITIS (EoE)

Eosinophilic esophagitis (EoE) is essentially "allergic esophagitis". It presents most commonly in people with allergic tendencies such as asthma, eczema, food allergy, and hay fever. It can also be associated with celiac disease. In adults, symptoms may include **dysphagia** or **impaction**, chest pain and regurgitation. In children the symptoms are more likely to be vomiting, pain and trouble eating enough food, which may lead to poor growth, malnutrition and weight loss commonly referred to as failure to thrive. Some cases respond to a trial of proton pump inhibitors.

Esophageal Motility Disorders

Esophageal motility disorders are problems with the coordination or strength of the muscles that move the bolus through the esophagus. **Achalasia, diffuse esophageal spasm** and **jackhammer esophagus** are examples of motility disorders.

Asthma and **GERD**

The clinical picture of GERD is varied but can include increased triggering of asthma symptoms (Amarasiri LD, 2010).

The relationship between asthma and GERD can be experienced by the patient as an aggravating cycle. While GERD can trigger asthma symptoms, medications used to treat asthma may in turn aggravate GERD. Those with asthma have twice the risk of experiencing GERD as those not diagnosed with asthma. According to the Cleveland Clinic website, up to 75% of people with asthma may also have GERD.

While GERD can trigger asthma symptoms, medications used to treat asthma may in turn aggravate GERD.

There are several theories to explain this relationship. The first is something called a vagal reflex, a response to the presence of acid or pressure from reflux in the esophagus. This reflex stimulates narrowing of the small airways in the lungs, a condition called bronchoconstriction, resulting in more asthma. Inhaling even a fine mist of gastric secretions (micro-aspiration) into the lungs may aggravate asthmatic breathing patterns. (Harding SM, 2013). Conversely, asthma may cause GERD. Asthmatic lungs may trigger a vagal reflex and GERD.

This chapter reviewed the types of reflux and causes of heartburn unrelated to reflux. All sorts of diseases and syndromes can coexist in the same person which makes the job of the physician so darn interesting!

In chapter three, we will go into detail regarding GERD, including the causes, both frequently diagnosed and less well known.

CITATIONS

Richter JE, Rubenstein JH, Presentation and Epidemiology of Gastroesophageal Reflux Disease. Gastroenterology. 2018;154(2): 267-276. PMID: 28780072

Delshad SD, Almario CV, Chey WD, Spiegel BMR, Prevalence of Gastroesophageal Reflux Disease and Proton Pump Inhibitor-Refractory Symptoms. Gastroenterology 2020 Apr; 158(5): 1250-1261.e2. PMID: 31866243

Friedman M et al, Measurements of adult lingual tonsil tissue in health and disease. Otolaryngol Head Neck Surg. 2010 Apr;142(4):520-5. PMID: 20304271

Amarasiri LD, Pathmeswaran A, de Siva HJ, Ranasinha CD, Prevalence of gastro-oesophageal reflux disease symptoms and reflux-associated respiratory symptoms in asthma. BMC Pulm Med. 2010 Sep 15;10:49. PMID: 20843346

Harding SM, Allen JE, Blumin JH, Warner EA et al, Respiratory manifestations of gastroesophageal reflux disease. Ann N Y Acad Sci. 2013 Oct;1300:43-52. PMID: 24117633

(https://my.clevelandclinic.org/health/articles/10686-gerd-and-asthma)

Yamasaki T, Fass R, Reflux Hypersensitivity: A New Functional Esophageal Disorder. J Neurogastroenterol Motil. 2017 Oct; 23(4): 495–503. PMID: 28992673

THREE

OVERVIEW OF CAUSES OF GERD

Reasons for GERD can be manyfold.
Don't blame it on being very old.
Transient relaxation,
Or the wrong medication,
And many more causes, you'll soon be told.

GLOSSARY

achalasia—a nerve disorder in which the LES cannot relax, causing obstruction and inability for food to enter the stomach

amyotrophic lateral sclerosis—a progressive nervous system disease that affects nerve cells in the brain and spinal cord, causing loss of muscle control

archaea—a family of intestinal organisms distinct from bacteria

autoimmune diseases—a group of diseases in which the immune system attacks one's own healthy cells

autonomic nervous system—the part of the nervous system responsible for control of the bodily functions not consciously directed, such as breathing, the heartbeat, and digestive processes

bariatric—referring to the study and treatment of obesity

Barrett's esophagus—a change in the type of cells lining the lower esophagus in response to chronic gastric reflux

barium swallow x-ray series—a diagnostic test comprised of a series of x-rays of the esophagus, stomach, and duodenum; also called an upper GI series

bile acids—components of bile, produced in the liver and stored in the gall bladder, that allow fat and water to mix

carcinogenic—having the potential to cause cancer

central obesity—an excess accumulation of fat in the abdominal area, surrounding the organs

chronic traumatic encephalopathy (CTE)—repeated episodes of brain trauma that lead to progressive dementia and loss of brain function

defensins—antibiotic proteins produced by white blood cells

diffuse esophageal spasm—an esophageal muscle disorder in which contractions are uncoordinated, painful and impede transport of food to the stomach

dilated intercellular spaces (DIS)—a widened microscopic space between esophageal mucosal cells. This is the esophageal version of "leaky gut"

gastric—of or pertaining to the stomach

gastric emptying study (gastric scintigraphy)—a diagnostic test which measures how long food remains in the stomach after a meal

gastroparesis—a disease in which the emptying of food from the stomach into the small intestine is slowed. Symptoms may include heartburn, nausea, vomiting, and feeling full quickly when eating

delayed gastric emptying—gastroparesis

hiatus—a gap or opening

high fermentation diet—a diet providing the gut microbiome with high amounts of carbohydrates which may allow the microbes to grow excessively and make excessive gas

hyperchlorhydria—excess production of gastric acid

hypochlorhydria—decreased production of gastric acid

hypermobility type Ehlers-Danlos syndrome—a genetic condition affecting collagen protein and resulting in unstable joint structures and lax internal organs

hyperosmolar—solutions that contain high levels of solutes such as minerals or sugars

intra-abdominal—within the abdomen

intrathoracic—within the chest

jackhammer esophagus—an esophageal dysmotility disorder in which contractions of high intensity cause chest pain

lactoferrin—an antioxidant, anti-inflammatory and antimicrobial protein that is found in milk, tears, mucus, bile, and saliva

lipopolysaccharide— a component of bacterial cell walls which triggers inflammation in the human body

lysozyme—an enzyme that acts as an antibiotic in body fluids such as breast milk, tears, and saliva

microbiome - microorganisms in a particular part of the body; in each part of the GI tract there is a unique mix of organisms —oral, esophageal, gastric, enteric, and colonic

mucosal blood flow—circulation in the blood vessels of the mucus membrane

multiple sclerosis—an autoimmune disease involving damage to the sheaths of nerve cells in the brain and spinal cord

non-steroidal anti-inflammatory drugs—pain and inflammation relieving medicines such as ibuprofen and naproxen

Parkinson's disease—a progressive disease of the nervous system marked by tremor, muscular rigidity, and slow, imprecise movements

rheumatoid arthritis—an autoimmune disease leading to joint deformity and inflammation of other tissues

scleroderma—an autoimmune disease which causes hardening and contraction of the skin and connective tissue, often affecting the esophagus as well as other organs; also referred to as progressive systemic sclerosis or CREST syndrome

secretory IgA—a protective antibody found in many body fluids

Sjogren's syndrome—autoimmune degeneration of the salivary and lachrymal glands, causing dryness of the mouth and eyes.

smart pill test—a diagnostic test which allows monitoring of pH and pressure throughout the entire GI tract.

steroid—fat soluble hormones derived from cholesterol

submucosal glands —glands deep to the esophageal mucosa that produce mucus and bicarbonate

systemic lupus (lupus erythematosus)—a multisystem autoimmune disease

terminal ileum—the last portion of the small intestine in which bile salts and B12 are absorbed

traumatic brain injuries (TBI)— a sudden trauma to the central nervous system which causes damage to the brain

trypsin—a protein digesting enzyme produced in the pancreas

type I diabetes—a form of diabetes marked by a deficiency of insulin production

KEY QUESTIONS

What substances are damaging to the esophagus?

How does the esophagus protect itself?

What are underlying mechanisms causing reflux?

In the first chapter I explained the structure and function of the GI tract with more focus on the esophagus, stomach, and duodenum. In Chapter Two, I explained that heartburn and gastroesophageal reflux, although they may overlap, are not the same thing. In this chapter I will discuss the important underlying mechanisms that allow GERD to occur.

These include:

1) Decreased levels of protective factors
2) Increased levels of potentially damaging factors
    a. acidic, weakly acidic and neutral reflux
    b. bile reflux
    c. drugs and lifestyle choices
3) Changes in esophageal muscle tone or coordination
    a. weakness of the lower esophageal sphincter muscle
    b. transient lower esophageal sphincter relaxations
    c. esophageal motility disorders
    d. delayed gastric emptying
4) Structural factors
    a. hiatal hernia
    b. the acid pocket
    c. gastric surgery
5) Increased pressure levels in the abdomen
6) Underhydration
7) Visceral hypersensitivity
8) Dilated intercellular spaces (DIS)

DECREASED LEVELS OF PROTECTIVE FACTORS

The esophagus has factors protecting it from the minimal amount of reflux of stomach contents normally occurring after meals. When the factors are in balance, GERD does not occur. This is physiological reflux as opposed to pathological. One of the major protective factors for the esophagus is saliva. As mentioned in the previous chapter, saliva is a big deal. The salivary glands normally produce over a liter of saliva per day. Healthy saliva is slightly alkaline (pH 7.5) which helps to neutralize any acid reflux that does occur. An autoimmune disease called **Sjogren's syndrome** often leads to GERD because it causes decreased salivation.

Saliva also contains **defensins, secretory IgA, lysozyme** and **lactoferrin**—all of which have a protective role for the lining of the esophagus. The esophagus, like the rest of the digestive tract, also produces mucus to lubricate and protect itself.

TABLE 3.1. ESOPHAGEAL PROTECTIVE FACTORS

Integrity of the esophageal mucosal cells

Saliva—contains alkaline buffers, defensins, SIgA, lysozyme, lactoferrin

Additional **bicarbonate** from **esophageal submucosal glands** neutralizes esophageal refluxed acid.

Mucus creates a barrier against the aggressive action of acid and pepsin.

The esophageal and gastric **microbiom**e interact with the mucus membrane.

Mucosal blood flow—adequate blood flow supplies oxygen and hormones controlling the local blood flow. This blood flow carries away excess acid. The blood flow increases during reflux events and brings in more bicarbonate to maintain an alkaline pH during episodes of reflux.

Melatonin—this potent antioxidant and GI hormone is one of the sundry factors protecting the mucosa and keeping gastric acid production in balance.

TABLE 3.2. ESOPHAGEAL AGGRESSIVE (POTENTIALLY DAMAGING) FACTORS

Gastric acid and pepsin are substances that can digest the layers of the esophageal wall.

Bile acids, trypsin, and **hyperosmolar** solutions (from duodenogastric reflux) can cause additional damage and may be carcinogenic.

Cigarette smoking, alcohol, **non-steroidal anti-inflammatory drugs** (NSAIDs) and **steroid** medications can damage the mucosa.

INCREASED LEVELS OF POTENTIALLY DAMAGING FACTORS

HYPERCHLORHYDRIA (TRUE EXCESS ACID PRODUCTION)

Acid and pepsin are in the stomach to digest protein. When these reflux into the esophagus they may trigger inflammation or erosion of the mucus membrane. In my practice, when testing those with heartburn, I use the Heidelberg radiotelemetry capsule test to directly measure the patient's gastric pH. The test is described in more detail in chapter four. Over the last four decades, I have found that about 20% of the population I have tested has **hyperchlorhydria.**

Because advertisements indoctrinate us with messages about excess stomach acid, it may be surprising to learn that about 60% of the heartburn patients I test have **hypochlorhydria** and only 20% have normal levels of acid.

WEAKLY ACIDIC AND NON-ACIDIC REFLUX (WAR)

The digestive enzyme pepsin is also in the chyme that refluxes from the stomach to the esophagus. It may cause symptoms or damage the esophagus even if the reflux has little or no acid.

Even if the refluxed material is not acidic, symptoms of reflux can occur. Studies show that just the pressure of refluxed material into the esophagus can cause burning or other types of chest pain. (Kondo T, 2017). Symptoms of reflux can occur when the stomach secretions are acidic, weakly acidic, or even mildly alkaline. Remember that the digestive enzyme pepsin is also in the chyme that refluxes from the stomach to the esophagus. It may cause symptoms or damage the esophagus even if the reflux has little or no acid.

BILE REFLUX

Health is all about balance. Bile belongs in the small intestine and minimally in the large intestine. After a meal containing fat, the gallbladder releases bile which flows through the entire 18-20 feet of small intestine and is then reabsorbed in the **terminal ileum**.

From the terminal ileum, components of the bile are absorbed into the blood and return to the liver to start the process all over again. Diseases of the terminal ileum (e.g., Crohn's disease) or surgical removal of the terminal ileum may reduce reabsorption of bile. If too much bile enters the large intestine, it acts as an irritant and can be a cause of severe diarrhea, referred to as bile acid diarrhea. Additionally, in irritable bowel syndrome, people may be ultrasensitive to normal amounts of bile in the colon.

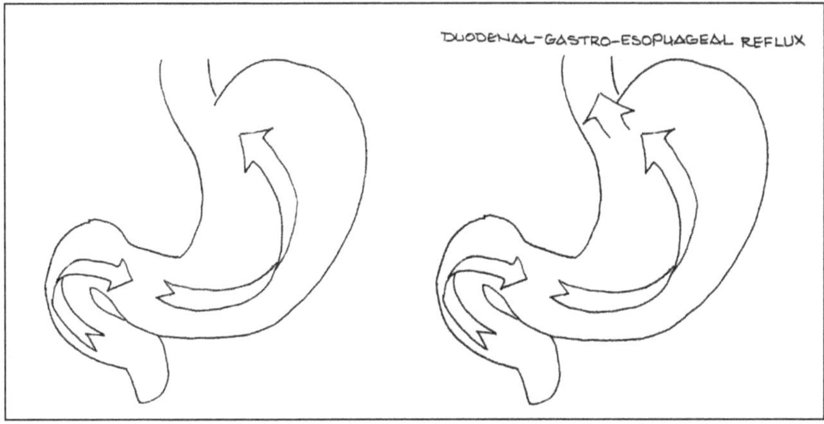

Fig. 3.1. Bile reflux (left) and DGER (right).

Sometimes bile flows upward into the stomach. This is called bile reflux and can cause an irritation of the stomach lining referred to as **bile gastritis**. Bile reflux occurs when the pyloric valve allows fluid from the duodenum to enter the stomach. If there is also GERD, the bile mixed with the stomach juices will reflux into the esophagus. This two-step reflux is called duodenal-gastro-esophageal reflux (DGER) or gastroesophageal bile reflux. Some researchers believe that the more severe complications of chronic reflux (such as Barrett's esophagus, Barrett's with dysplasia and esophageal adenocarcinoma) may be related to this type of process rather than merely gastroesophageal reflux alone (Wolfgarten E, 2007). Acid suppressive medicines are less effective for DGER than for GERD (Tack J, 2004). Bile reflux is more common in patients with more severe grades of erosive esophagitis (Monaco L, 2009).

DRUGS AND LIFESTYLE CHOICES

Over the counter and prescription medications can trigger or lead to GERD. For example, a common group of prescription drugs for osteoporosis called bisphosphonates commonly cause or increase heartburn and esophagitis. Examples of these include alendronate (Fosamax), risedronate (Actonel) and ibandronate (Boniva). Due to this relationship, injectable medications that bypass the digestive tract and do not trigger esophageal irritation are also available for treatment of osteoporosis.

Lifestyle choices that promote GERD are discussed in chapter eight.

CHANGES IN ESOPHAGEAL MUSCLE TONE OR COORDINATION

WEAKNESS OF THE LOWER ESOPHAGEAL SPHINCTER MUSCLE

The lower esophageal sphincter (LES), a thickened portion of the esophageal smooth muscle layer, is essential for controlling the movement of food from the esophagus into the stomach, and once there, keeping the stomach contents from returning to the esophagus. Ideally, the LES opens when the wave of peristalsis triggered by swallowing food or liquid reaches the lower esophagus. When working properly, the LES opens momentarily and then closes again after the bolus passes into the stomach. If this coordination is not perfect or if the LES muscle is weak, various terms are used to describe the problem. These include LES laxity and reduced LES tone.

To function properly, the LES must be surrounded by the diaphragm, which is the large, thin muscle that separates the chest from the abdomen. The diaphragm has tendons called the left crus and right crus, which means leg. These crura encircle the

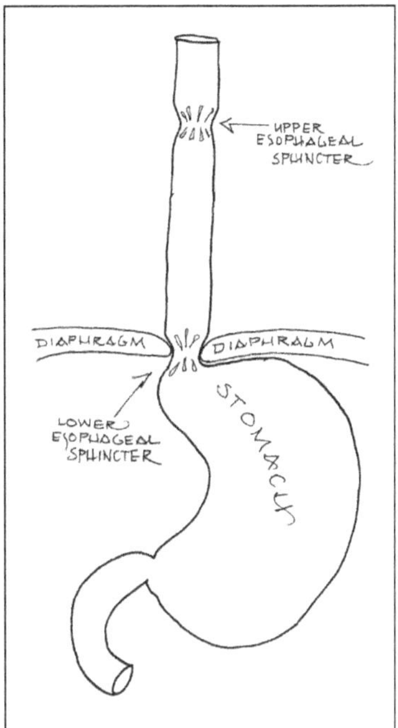

Fig. 3.2. Upper and lower esophageal sphincters.

To function properly, the LES must be surrounded by the diaphragm.

The diaphram encircles the esophagus at the level of the LES.

esophagus at the level of the LES as shown in Fig 3.2. They form the **hiatus** of the diaphragm with the esophagus above and stomach below. In the sport of wrestling, "scissors hold" describes a maneuver in which one wrestler wraps their legs around their opponent's neck. This is the shape of the crura in relationship to the esophagus. Although the diaphragm and esophagus are separate structures, you might think of the diaphragm as an outer supporting layer of the LES muscle. If the diaphragm has poor tone or isn't lined up properly with the LES, reflux is more likely.

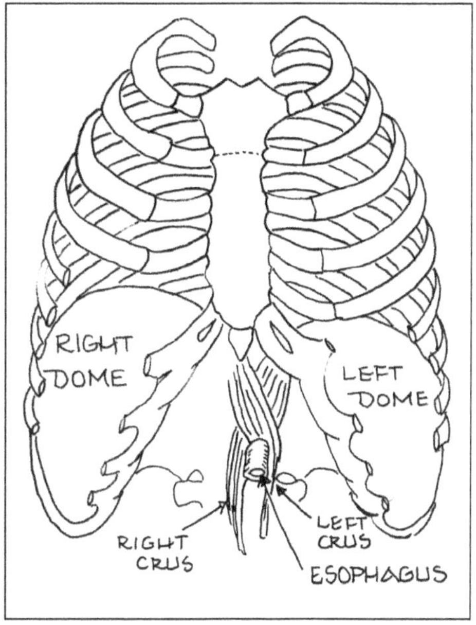

Fig. 3.3. Relationships among diaphragm, ribs, and esophagus.

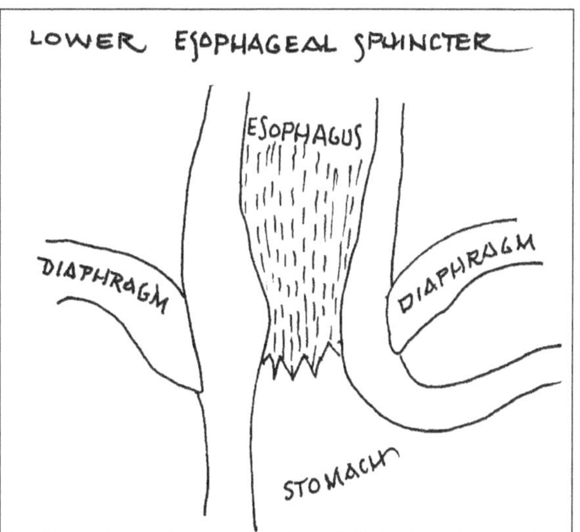

Fig. 3.4. Cross section with relationships among diaphragm, esophagus, and stomach.

Asthma medications may decrease the tone of the lower esophageal sphincter and cause GERD. Examples of such drugs include beta-agonists, such albuterol (Ventolin, Proventil), metaproterenol (Alupent), pirbuterol (Maxair), terbutaline (Brethaire), isoetharine (Bronkosol), levalbuterol (Xopenex) and salmeterol (Serevent).

Some medications prescribed for heart problems and high blood pressure can also weaken the LES. These include nitrates such as isosorbide mononitrate (Imdur, Monoket) and dinitrate (Isordil), as well as calcium channel blockers such as amlodipine (Norvasc), diltiazem (Cardizem), felodipine (Plendil), nicardipine (Cardene), and nifedipine (Adalat, Procardia). Additional drugs that can weaken the LES muscle tone include some diarrhea medications (anticholinergics such as atropine in Lomotil), narcotics, and sedatives such as benzodiazepines and barbiturates (Cleveland Clinic website).

TRANSIENT LOWER ESOPHAGEAL SPHINCTER RELAXATIONS (TLESRs)

Reflux also occurs during transient lower esophageal sphincter relaxations (TLESRs) which happen for a variety of reasons. (Refer to chapter one for discussion of the normal process of swallowing and the relaxation of the LES.)

In the case of TLESRs, the relaxation of the LES is not associated with swallowing. These relaxations are triggered by distension caused by excessive pressure from solid, liquid or gas in the stomach and enable gas to vent from the stomach through the LES, into the esophagus and out the mouth. Gas can also move down the intestinal tract, causing flatulence, but that route does not create reflux.

TLESRs last for about 20 seconds, which is significantly longer than the typical relaxation induced by swallowing. If these occur frequently or have longer duration, they are another risk factor for GERD.

ESOPHAGEAL MOTILITY DISORDERS

Motility disorders are diseases in which the coordinated patterns of muscles in the esophagus are abnormal. These include **scleroderma, diffuse esophageal spasm, jackhammer esophagus and achalasia.** Abnormal esophageal function can also occur in **neurological diseases such as Parkinson's and amyotrophic lateral**

sclerosis (ALS). Some patients develop changes in esophageal muscle function as long as two years after a thyroidectomy, which is surgery to remove the thyroid gland, (Scerrino G, 2017 and Danic-Hadzibegovic A, 2020).

DELAYED GASTRIC EMPTYING (GASTROPARESIS)

Gastroparesis is the partial paralysis of the stomach muscles. There are several possible causes of gastroparesis:

- Diabetes—
    Occurs in 55-75% of type 1 diabetics
    Occurs in 15-20% of type 2 diabetics
- Lupus
- Hypothyroidism
- Scleroderma
- Parkinson's
- Stroke
- Traumatic brain injury
- Drug side effects:
    Tobacco
    Calcium channel blockers
    L-dopa
    Hyoscyamine
    Anticholinergics
    Opiates

Delayed gastric emptying is diagnosed when more than 10% of chyme is still in the stomach four or more hours after a meal.

Delayed gastric emptying occurs when more than 10% of chyme is still in the stomach four or more hours after a meal. Many medications slow gastric emptying. Some of the more common drugs with this side effect include tobacco, calcium channel blockers, L-dopa, hyoscyamine, anticholinergics and narcotics. It is also suspected that people with **hypermobility type Ehlers-Danlos syndrome** are also more prone to have delayed emptying (Alomari M, 2020). Nerve injury from traumatic brain injury or viral illness can also lead to gastroparesis.

Symptoms often include heartburn, regurgitation of food into the throat, excessive burping, the sensation of being full after small portions of food, nausea, vomiting, and upper abdominal cramping.

The most common way to test for gastroparesis is to perform a **gastric emptying study** (gastric scintigraphy). A "smart" **pill test** or a **barium swallow x-ray series** are less commonly used ways to diagnose gastroparesis.

Structural Factors

Hiatal Hernia

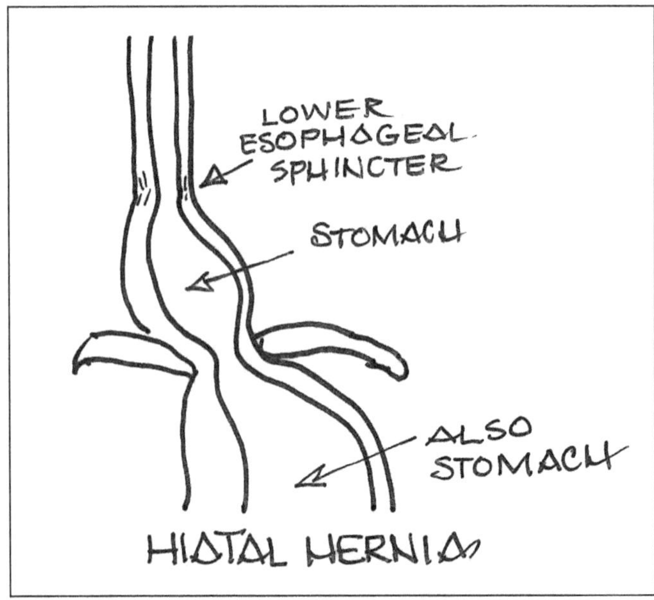

Fig. 3.5. Hiatal hernia.

A hiatal hernia occurs when the upper portion of the stomach rises into the chest.

This makes GERD more likely.

A hiatal hernia occurs when the upper portion of the stomach rises into the chest, disengaging the diaphragm from the LES and causing the LES to lose tone, making GERD more likely when this happens. Hiatal hernia and its related syndrome will be discussed in more detail in chapter thirteen.

Acid Pocket

"Acid pocket" describes the natural accumulation of stomach acid in the fundus, making the top of the stomach the most acidic part. Accumulation of acid so close to the LES may facilitate reflux. The longer the pocket persists, its length and increasing acidity are significantly associated with acid exposure in the esophagus (Wu J. 2018).

Having a hiatal hernia along with a significant acid pocket increases reflux via several mechanisms (Kahrilas PJ, 2013). Acid pocket is a factor in Barrett's esophagus, a chronic complication of reflux (Nyan YY, 2020).

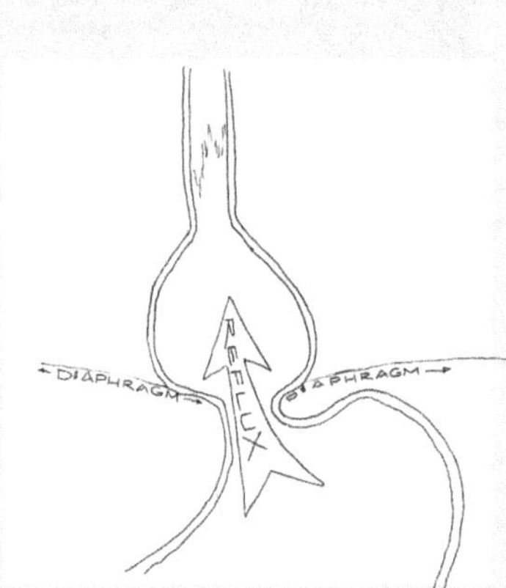

Fig. 3.6. Hiatal hernia with acid pocket.

In the chapter on natural treatments for reflux, I will discuss a gel-based treatment to address acid pocket.

Gastric Surgery

Laparoscopic sleeve gastrectomy (LSG) is a **bariatric** surgery that frequently leads to increased intragastric pressure (Mion F et al, 2016). Research has shown that although LSG may help improve GERD in 25% of those patients who had GERD prior to the surgery, it may also *cause* the onset of GERD in 10–31% of patients (Juodeikis Z 2017). It can also cause the stomach to migrate into the chest, creating a hiatal hernia (Termine P, 2021). Further research has shown that during the five years following LSG, the incidence of GERD, erosive esophagitis and use of proton pump inhibitors increases significantly. Over 17% of these patients develop **Barrett's esophagus**, which is a complication of long-term reflux (Sebastianelli L, 2019).

Increased Pressure Levels in the Abdomen

People often mistakenly refer to the entire abdomen as the "stomach", but the term stomach refers to the organ just below the esophagus.

The respiratory diaphragm divides the trunk of the body into the chest and the abdomen. Everything above the diaphragm is thoracic, referring to the chest, and everything below the diaphragm is abdominal. The pressure in the chest is called **intrathoracic** pressure. The pressure in the abdomen is called **intra-abdominal** pressure.

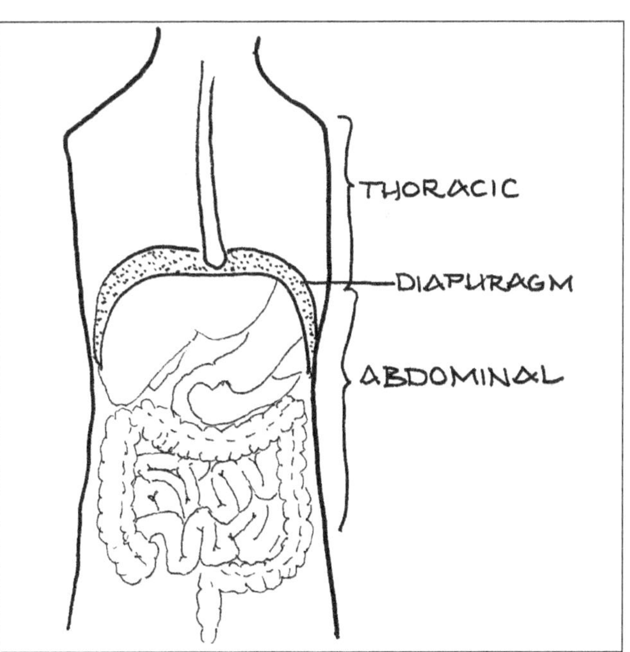

Fig. 3.7. Thoracic and abdominal cavities.

People often mistakenly refer to the entire abdomen as the "stomach", but the term stomach refers to the organ just below the esophagus. The adjective referring to the stomach is **"gastric"** as in the word gastroesophageal—which means stomach and esophagus.

Reflux can occur when increases in intra-abdominal pressure (pressure levels below the diaphragm) overpower the LES. Increased abdominal pressure may occur with **central obesity** (also referred to as "apple fat"), pregnancy, delayed gastric emptying, overeating, constipation with build-up of stool in the large intestine, and breath holding.

Breath holding, a common tendency, significantly increases abdominal pressure especially if done while straining, such as during a bowel movement or weightlifting, which causes the abdominal muscles to contract. Breath holding is discussed further in the chapter entitled "Your Brain May Be Sabotaging Your Digestion". Breath holding is also referred to as the "Valsalva maneuver" in healthcare terms. Inhaling and then holding the breath during exertion seems to create the highest pressures in the abdomen. Both lax LES tone and the presence of a hiatal hernia increase the risk of reflux episodes during periods of increased intra-abdominal pressure.

Breath holding significantly increases intra-abdominal pressure.

Another common cause of increased intra-abdominal pressure is excessive gas distending the small intestine. Most intestinal gases, such as hydrogen or methane, are produced when carbohydrate foods are processed by bacteria and other microorganisms. The term "fermentation" refers to this process, whether occurring internally by bacteria in the intestine or externally by yeast in a barrel during the production of alcoholic beverages or by lactic acid bacteria in the making of sauerkraut. Some diets contain more carbohydrates for these organisms to turn into gas and may be referred to as high fermentation diets.

A diet high in fermentable carbohydrates is another cause of increased intra-abdominal pressure.

Certain foods are more fermentable, such as grains, whole milk, beans, onions, and garlic. Besides a high fermentation diet, an overgrowth of the microorganisms in the small intestine will also create more gas and pressure. This is called Small Intestine Bacterial Overgrowth or intestinal methanogen overgrowth (SIBO or IMO). See chapter sixteen for more on these conditions. SIBO is associated with many diseases, including erosive esophagitis.

Underhydration

The adult human body is approximately 60% water.

Saliva is 99% water and dilutes physiological reflux.

Heartburn can be the result of the inadequate intake of water and electrolytes. According to the US Geological Survey, the adult human body is approximately 60% water. Salivary glands make up to 1.5 liters of saliva per day which is mostly water (99%). With decreased water intake, there is less saliva production. Also of note is that saliva is swallowed every minute all through the day. This process bathes the esophagus in neutral or slightly alkaline fluid because healthy saliva has a pH of 7.0-7.5 which protects the esophagus and dilutes any physiological reflux from the stomach.

While moderate intensity exercise is beneficial in many ways, overtraining or strenuous exercise may trigger heartburn and other digestive system problems due, in part, to underhydration. Moderate intensity exercise, with proper hydration, helps to protect against colon cancer, diverticular disease, gallstones, and constipation. (Prado de Oliveira E, 2009).

Visceral Hypersensitivity

Visceral hypersensitivity may be best treated with bio-feedback, self-hypnosis and mindfulness.

Visceral hypersensitivity, the perception of pain in response to normal pressures or muscular activity in the gut, is a tough situation. It is not easy to treat and may be best addressed through the nervous system. It often requires biofeedback, self-hypnosis and/or mindfulness practices to calm the nervous system and increase the "rest and digest" portion of the **autonomic nervous system**. You will find more about the autonomic nervous system in chapter eleven.

Patients with reflux hypersensitivity have heartburn symptoms that are related to physiological reflux. They do not have pathological GERD, as determined by pH impedance monitoring. The current theory is that this type of heartburn is related to visceral hypersensitivity causing the perception of pain or burning from the normal activity taking place in the esophagus. Visceral hypersensitivity has been found to be associated with nerve inflammation in those with NERD (Yoshida N, 2013).

Dilated Intercellular Spaces (DIS)—
The Esophageal Version of "Leaky Gut"

Most people have heard of "leaky gut", a well-researched phenomenon but, for the details, an explanation is given in the grey box at the end of this chapter.

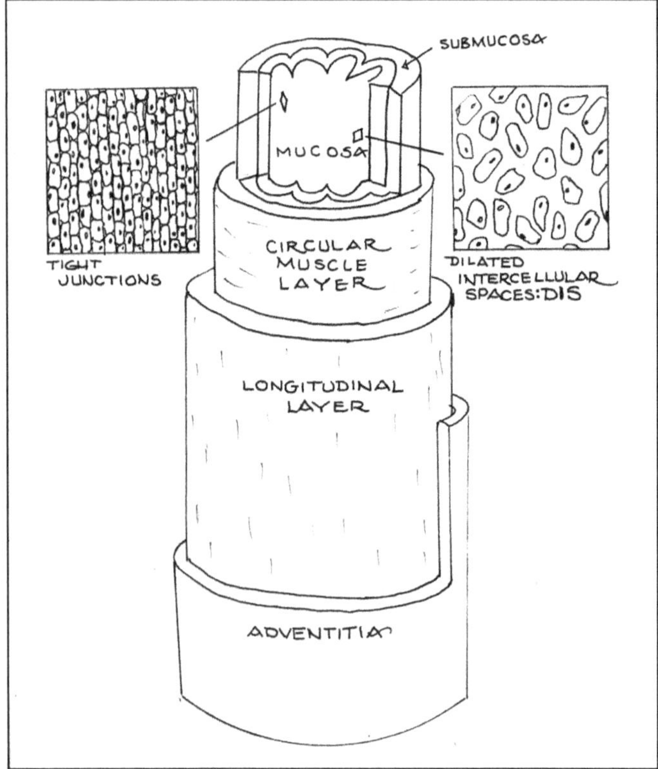

Fig. 3.8. Microscopic appearance of dilated intercellular spaces.

A condition like leaky gut can occur in the stomach and esophagus. Within the esophagus it is called dilated intercellular spaces (DIS). The microscopic spaces between individual squamous cells that line the mucus membrane of the inner esophagus have important protective effects. This area between cells is not merely open space. Instead, it is traversed by microscopic protein bridge-like structures called intercellular junctional complexes. When these bridges are damaged by chronic reflux, the space widens which may allow the nerves and blood vessels in the deeper lining of the esophagus to be irritated. DIS may be an explanation for why even weakly acidic reflux can cause reflux symptoms. Most patients with GERD and 30% of those without GERD have DIS. DIS is diagnosed for research purposes using upper endoscopy with biopsy. It is not reported on standard diagnostic esophageal biopsy reports because it requires a special electron microscope to reveal such detail, but it has been well described in the research literature (Orlando LA, 2009). Some studies have shown that treatment with proton pump inhibitors may normalize DIS in GERD patients (Kahrilas PJ, 2005).

What Is a Leaky Gut?

Intestinal hyperpermeability is commonly referred to as "leaky gut". The normal function of the intestines, particularly the small intestine, is to absorb properly digested food into the bloodstream. The epithelial cells making up the mucus membrane of the small intestine have finger-like projections called villi. Villi are part of what creates the huge surface area needed for absorption of nutrients. The surface area of the small intestinal lining is about 2,700 square feet. This massive absorptive lining also serves as a barrier to keep the intestinal bacteria and other organisms inside the intestines and out of the blood. In addition, it is the interface at which everything moving through the digestive tract interacts with the largest portion of the immune system.

In between adjacent lining cells is a space called the tight junction. It has several complex parts, but it is a microscopic space that normally permits only the smallest molecules to pass through. When the mucus membrane becomes inflamed the tight junctions can become "loose" or "leaky" from the following:

- exposure to too much alcohol

- irritation from drugs such as ibuprofen or steroid medications

- celiac disease

- stress leading to excess cortisol levels

- **traumatic brain injuries** (TBI) and **chronic traumatic encephalopathy** (CTE)

An imbalance in the intestinal microbiome (bacteria, yeast, viruses, and other organisms in the gut) can also trigger the gut lining to become more permeable. This can alter the ways that food and intestinal organisms interact with the immune system and even allow some of the bacteria or the irritating substances they produce to enter the blood or lymph systems. One example of this is **lipopolysaccharide** (LPS). When this bacterial-made substance gets absorbed into the blood, it can trigger immune reactions throughout the body. There is further evidence that these reactions are involved in autoimmune diseases including type I diabetes, systemic lupus, rheumatoid arthritis, and multiple sclerosis (Ilchmann-Diounou H, 2020).

Now that you have a foundation for understanding the mechanisms that lead to GERD, we will discuss how to properly test for GERD and other GI issues.

CITATIONS

Ilchmann-Diounou H, Menard S, Psychological Stress, Intestinal Barrier Dysfunctions, and Autoimmune Disorders: An Overview, Front Immunol . 2020 Aug 25;11:1823. PMID: 32983091

Orlando LA, Orlando RC. Dilated intercellular spaces as a marker of GERD. Curr Gastroenterol Rep. 2009 Jun;11(3):190-4. PMID: 19463218

Kahrilas PJ, Dilated intercellular spaces: extending the reach of the endoscope. Am J Gastroenterol. 2005 Mar;100(3):549-50. PMID: 15743350

Scerrino G, Tudisca C, Bonvnetre S, Raspanti C, et al. Swallowing disorders after thyroidectomy: What we know and where we are. A systematic review. Int J Surg. 2017 May;41 Suppl 1:S94-S102. PMID: 28506421

Danic Hadzibegovic A, Hergesic F, Babic E, Slipac J, Thyroidectomy-related Swallowing Difficulties: Review of the Literature. Acta Clin Croat. 2020 Jun;59 (Suppl 1):38-49. PMID: 34219883

Alomari M, Hitawala A, Chadalavada P, Covut F, et al. Prevalence and Predictors of Gastrointestinal Dysmotility in Patients with Hypermobile Ehlers-Danlos Syndrome: A Tertiary Care Center Experience. Cureus. 2020 Apr 29;12(4):e7881. PMID: 32489735

Suri J, Kataria R, Malik Z, Parkman HP et al, Elevated methane levels in small intestinal bacterial overgrowth suggests delayed small bowel and colonic transit. Medicine (Baltimore). 2018 May; 97(21): e10554. PMID: 29794732

Pimentel M, Lin HC, Enayati P, van den Burg B, Lee HR, Chen JH, et al. Methane, a gas produced by enteric bacteria, slows intestinal transit and augments small intestinal contractile activity. Am J Physiol Gastrointest Liver Physiol (2006) 290(6):G1089–95.

Wolfgarten E et al, Duodeno-Gastric-Esophageal Reflux—What is Pathologic? Comparison of Patients with Barrett's Esophagus and Age-Matched Volunteers, J Gastrointest Surg 2007 Apr; 11(4): 479–486. PMID: 17436133

Tack J et al, Gastroesophageal reflux disease poorly responsive to single-dose proton pump inhibitors in patients without Barrett's esophagus: acid reflux, bile reflux, or both? Am J Gastroenterol. 2004 Jun;99(6):981-8.

Monaco L et al, Prevalence of bile reflux in gastroesophageal reflux disease patients not responsive to proton pump inhibitors, World J Gastroenterol. 2009 Jan 21;15(3):334-8.

Boeckxstaens G, et al, The Relationship Between the Acid Pocket and GERD. Gastroenterol Hepatol (N.Y.) 2013 Sep; 9(9): 595–596. PMID: 24729769

Mion F et al, High-resolution Impedance Manometry after Sleeve Gastrectomy: Increased Intragastric Pressure and Reflux are Frequent Events. Obes Surg. 2016;26:2449–2456. PMID: 26956879

Termine P, Boru CE, Lossa A, Ciccioriccio MC, Transhiatal Migration After Laparoscopic Sleeve Gastrectomy: Myth or Reality? A Multicenter, Retrospective Study on the Incidence and Clinical Impact. Obes Surg. 2021 Aug;31(8):3419-3426.

Juodeikis Ž, Brimas G. Long-term results after sleeve gastrectomy: A systematic review. Surg Obes Relat Dis. 2017;13:693–699. PMID: 27876332

Sebastianelli L et al, Systematic Endoscopy 5 Years After Sleeve Gastrectomy Results in a High Rate of Barrett's Esophagus: Results of a Multicenter Study. Obes Surg. 2019;29:1462–1469. PMID: 30666544.

Kondo T, Miwa H, The Role of Esophageal Hypersensitivity in Functional Heartburn. J Clin Gastroenterol. 2017 Aug;51(7):571-578. PMID: 28682989

Wu J et al, The Characteristics of Postprandial Proximal Gastric Acid Pocket in Gastroesophageal Reflux Disease. Med Sci Monit 2018; 24: 170-176. PMID: 29309401

Kahrilas PJ et al, The acid pocket: a target for treatment in reflux disease? Am J Gastroenterol. 2013 Jul;108(7):1058-64. PMID: 23629599

Nyan YY et al, Postprandial proximal gastric acid pocket and its association with gastroesophageal acid reflux in patients with short-segment Barrett's esophagus. J Zhejiang Univ Sci B 2020 Jul; 21(7): 581–589. PMID: 32633112

Prado de Oliveira E, Carlos Burini R, Curr Opin Clin Nutr Metab Care. The impact of physical exercise on the gastrointestinal tract. 2009 Sep;12(5):533-8.

Yoshida N, Kuroda M, Suzuki T, Kamada K, et al. Role of nociceptors/neuropeptides in the pathogenesis of visceral hypersensitivity of nonerosive reflux disease. Dig Dis Sci. 2013 Aug;58(8):2237-43. PMID: 22899239

FOUR

Is It GERD?
Definitive Tests for Gastroesophageal Reflux Disease

Don't assume burning means you have GERD,
To take that for granted's absurd,
If acid suppression,
has taught any lesson,
A real test is vastly preferred.

Glossary

DeMeester score—a number calculated from the results of a pH impedance or Bravo capsule test

esophagogastroduodenoscopy (EGD)—a diagnostic scope exam used to examine the esophagus, stomach, and duodenum

esophagram—a series of x-ray pictures of the esophagus after a patient drinks a liquid solution of barium. This is a more focused test than the upper GI series discussed below

euchlorhydria—a normal level of stomach acid

radiolabeled—addition of a radioactive substance to a diagnostic test to allow accurate measurements

upper endoscopy—an alternate term for esophagogastroduodenoscopy or EGD

upper GI series—sometime called a "barium swallow" this group of diagnostic pictures examines the esophagus, stomach, and duodenum made visible on X-ray by a liquid suspension of barium

KEY QUESTIONS

What are the advanced tests for correctly diagnosing reflux and its complications?

Should symptom relief from a trial of a PPI be considered a diagnosis of reflux?

What are the Cytosponge and EsoGuard, and how might they revolutionize screening?

Problems Occur from Lack of Testing

Many who suffer from heartburn have not had tests that definitively diagnose GERD. Although the tests exist, the standard medical approach is to presume a diagnosis of GERD based on reported symptoms alone. This assumption is followed by writing a prescription for an acid blocking medication. This is often referred to as a proton pump inhibitor (PPI) trial. PPIs in various potencies are used to see if they will assuage symptoms.

Table 4.1. Proton Pumps and Proton Pump Inhibitors
Definitions: Proton pumps are microscopic structures within parietal cells located in the lining of the stomach. They produce and release hydrochloric acid. Proton pump inhibitors (PPIs) are pharmaceuticals that target proton pumps, minimizing (inhibiting) the release of that acid.
Side effects of proton pump inhibitors: • Hypergastrinemia—High levels of gastrin in the blood which may be a risk factor for gastric and colonic polyps or cancer. • Reduced absorption of calcium and magnesium which may lead to bone fracture (Koyyada A, 2021 and Liu J, 2019), muscle cramps or cardiac arrhythmias. Reduced absorption of iron and B12 may cause anemia (Fashner J, 2013). • Increased risk for bacterial or fungal overgrowth in the intestines. Overgrowth may cause digestive symptoms such as excess gas, bloating, abdominal pain, constipation or diarrhea, fatigue and anemia (Erdogan A, 2015). The overgrowth of *Clostridium difficile*, recently renamed *Clostridioides difficile* (abbreviation is *C. difficile*) is a form of severe bacterial diarrhea related to taking antibiotics. The risk of getting this disease while hospitalized is even higher if the patient is taking PPIs (Arriola V, 2016). • Increased risk for pneumonia - PPI use is associated with a 1.5-fold increased risk of pneumonia. The highest risk occurs in the first 30 days of taking the PPI (Lambert AA, 2015). • Increased risk for kidney disease (Wei X, 2022 and Vengrus CS, 2021)
The list of researched associations between PPI use and diseases goes beyond the details in this section. Multiple meta-analyses as well as systems for grading the quality of the PPI research have been used to try to clarify association versus causation. Except for the increased risk for magnesium deficiency and *C. difficile* diarrhea, most of these complications of long-term PPI use are hotly debated.

Often, people have told me that they have been to their primary care physicians with the symptom of heartburn and come home with a prescription for proton pump inhibitors.

Specialty tests for GERD are not part of a primary care physician's toolkit. Such specific tests are performed by gastroenterologists, when treatment trials have failed or when the patient's symptoms suggest more serious disease. The definitive tests become standard only when the option of reflux surgery is investigated. No surgeon wants to perform reflux surgery on someone who doesn't have reflux.

These tests are a good option when the patient is not respond-ing to standard treatment. The technology allows the gastroen-terologist to know whether the heartburn is truly a sign of reflux or something else. The tests may reveal important details about underlying causes such as LES laxity, the pH of the refluxed mate-rial, the presence of bile reflux, etc.

Jumping from unconfirmed diagnosis to daily proton pump inhibitor use sets the patient up for the possibility of side effects and complications from a prescription that may not be appropri-ate for the condition.

This currently condoned approach of symptom management for what is presumed to be reflux often leads to a whack-a-mole approach to medicine. Too often I have seen patients with histories such as the following: A patient is prescribed omeprazole, a com-mon PPI, to suppress symptoms that sound as if they are related to GERD. Over time, the patient develops the PPI complication of pneumonia, which is then treated with antibiotics and ibuprofen. The latter drugs can cause esophageal and gastric inflammation. Additionally, PPIs frequently cause magnesium deficiency which may elevate blood pressure which will lead to a prescription for anti-hypertensive medication such as amlodipine. Amlodipine is a calcium channel blocker which has the potential to increase acid reflux and worsen GERD. PPIs are also associated with advancing osteoporosis which may be treated with alendronate, a bisphos-phonate known to irritate the esophagus and increase heartburn.

The above scenario begins with a good hunch on the part of the doctor ("these symptoms sure sound like reflux") but can lead to a self-fulfilling prophecy. The treatment eventually causes reflux as well as other new problems.

SPECIALTY TESTS FOR GERD

ENDOSCOPY

One study that can be performed is an **esophagogastroduodenos-copy (EGD)** known more commonly as an **upper endoscopy**. This involves sedation to allow a camera at the end of a small scope to be inserted into the mouth and advanced into the upper digestive tract as shown in the illustration. The camera can directly visualize the tissue lining the esophagus, stomach, and part of the duodenum (the first part of the small intestine).

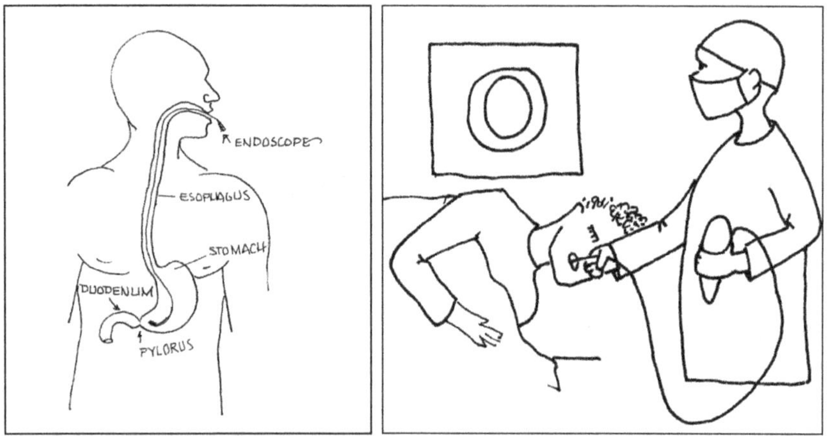

Fig. 4.1. The path of the upper endoscopy.   Fig. 4.2. Doctor performing upper endoscopy.

An upper endoscopy involves a narrow scope inserted into the mouth and extended as far as the duodenum.

An EGD allows the gastroenterologist to detect tissue affected by inflammation, ulcers, strictures, webs, rings, tears, or masses. During the procedure, certain corrective treatments may be performed, and samples of tissue can be biopsied for examination under a microscope. These biopsies may reveal diseases such as eosinophilic esophagitis, Barrett's esophagus, dysplasia, or cancer. The upper endoscopy results may be normal in patients with GERD. In fact, 40-60% of patients with GERD will have a normal endoscopic exam, termed non-erosive reflux disease (NERD). Alternately, there may be evidence of erosive esophagitis, which can be graded based on the severity. See Fig 4.3. and Table 4.2.

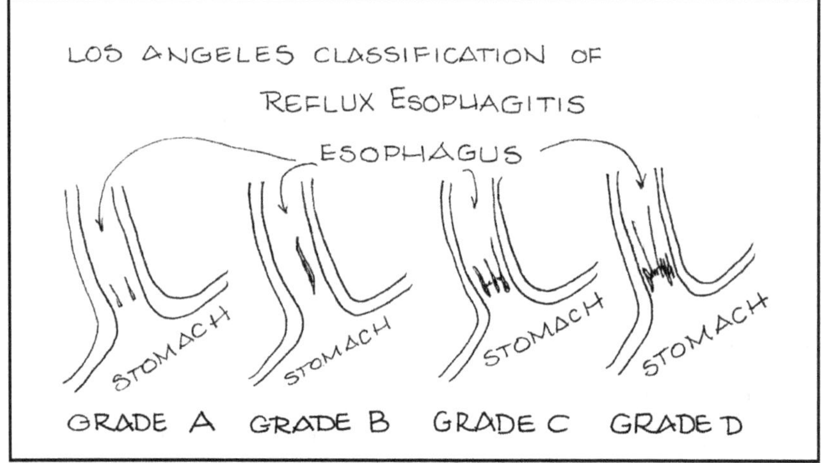

Fig. 4.3. LA reflux esophagitis grading system.

<table>
<tr><td colspan="1" align="center">TABLE 4.2. FOUR GRADES OF EROSIVE ESOPHAGITIS.</td></tr>
<tr><td>

- Grade A: One or more mucosal breaks confined to the mucosal folds, each not more than 5 mm in maximum length.

- Grade B: One or more mucosal breaks more than 5 mm in maximum length, but not continuous between the tops of two mucosal folds.

- Grade C: Mucosal breaks that are continuous between the tops of two or more mucosal folds, but which involve less than 75% of the esophageal circumference.

- Grade D: Mucosal breaks which involve at least 75% of the esophageal circumference.

</td></tr>
<tr><td>Source: www.ncbi.nlm.nih.gov/books/NBK47264/</td></tr>
</table>

CYTOSPONGE AND ESOGUARD
NEW, LESS INVASIVE SCREENINGS FOR BARRETT'S ESOPHAGUS (BE)

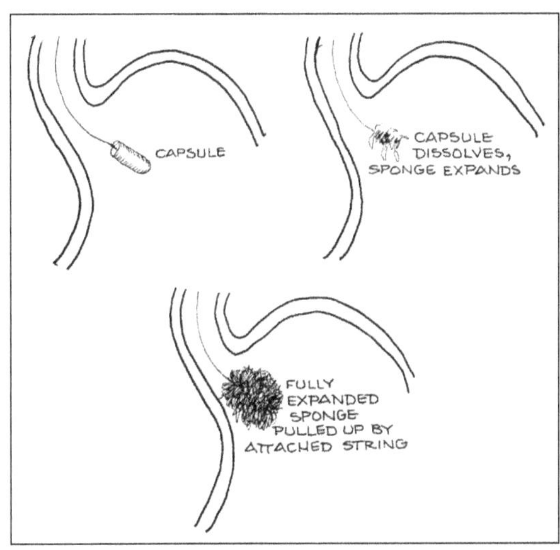

Fig. 4.4. Cytosponge screening for Barrett's esophagus.

The Cytosponge, already in use in the United Kingdom, and the EsoCheck and EsoCap are in development for use in the United States to screen for BE and esophageal cancer. EsoGuard is a more sophisticated device, already available in the United States, that enlarges when inflated, rather than using a sponge. All of these tests are designed for in-office use and do not require sedation. Similar to a PAP smear, these tests brush cells from body tissues to allow testing of cellular material.

Procedure for Cytosponge: A small thin sponge is packed into a capsule and attached to a string. As the capsule is swallowed, the string unwinds down into the stomach. The capsule dissolves rapidly, the sponge opens and is then pulled up through the esophagus. During this process the sponge gathers cells and DNA which can be analyzed by pathologists for the presence of Barrett's cells, dysplasia and a gene mutation that increases the risk of progression from BE to adenocarcinoma (Duits LC, 2019).

Procedure for EsoGuard: A thin plastic catheter is advanced from the mouth to the lower esophagus. The lower tip is inflated slightly and pulled through the lower esophagus. It is then deflated and removed for DNA testing as with the Cytosponge.

24-hour Combined Multichannel Intraluminal Impedance with pH testing (pH Impedance Monitoring)

This test monitors the amount and duration of reflux, both acidic and non-acidic, in the esophagus during a 24-hour period and shows whether symptoms correlate with reflux. It detects fluid moving upward in the esophagus, if present, and reveals how high the refluxed material travels. In most cases, the patient discontinues taking any acid suppressive medications for a week or two prior to the test.

Procedure: A thin flexible catheter is placed through one nostril and the patient swallows a little water to guide the catheter into the esophagus. The top end of the probe is taped to the cheek, wrapped over the ear, and attached to a data recorder worn at waist level. The recorder measures the frequency and pH of any reflux events while the patient records when they experience heartburn or reflux symptoms. This is done over a 24-hour period. When the data is examined, it will become clear whether reflux events are related to symptoms, helping to differentiate functional heartburn from symptoms of true reflux. It also allows differentiation among reflux that is acidic, weakly acidic, neutral, or alkaline. The results are used to calculate a **DeMeester score**. A normal DeMeester score is less than 14.72. Higher readings are determined to be mild, moderate, or severe GERD. (www.mdapp.com)

The **BRAVO** Test

A BRAVO test is similar to the pH impedance study, but only measures pH changes. It will fail to detect nonacid reflux. Some gastroenterologists find this to be a better initial test. The BRAVO test uses a pH measuring device in the lower esophagus that is mostly imperceptible to the patient, unlike the pH impedance monitor which involves a nasal catheter. Although the pH impedance test is able to detect more types of reflux, the catheter shown in Fig 4.5 will often inhibit normal activities and lifestyle factors that might make it less likely to accurately detect the patient's degree of reflux. The BRAVO also tests over a 48 hour period, whereas the pH impedance is a 24 hour test. Some patients do not have reflux daily, so a two day test may be beneficial. If the BRAVO does not indicate reflux, the pH impedance can be used as a second test.

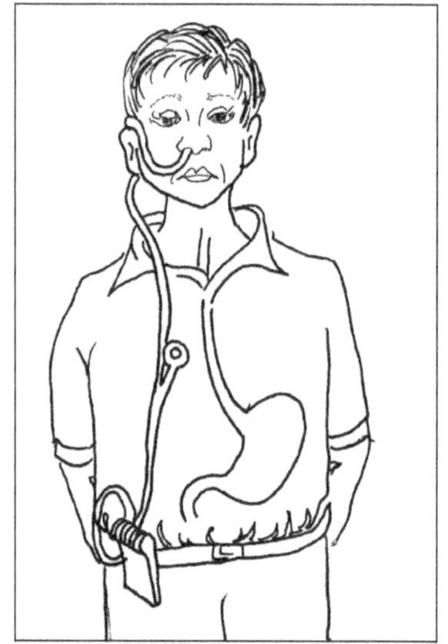

Fig. 4.5. 24-hour combined multi-channel intraluminal impedance with pH monitoring device.

The pH Impedance Monitor measures the frequency and pH of reflux events.

The Bravo test measures only acid reflux events.

A normal De Meester score is less than 14.72.

ESOPHAGEAL MANOMETRY

This is another test which is useful in evaluating the movement and flexibility of the esophagus. It evaluates pressure and coordination of muscular contractions as well as the tone/strength of the upper and lower esophageal sphincters.

Procedure: A small diameter tube is passed through the nose and into the esophagus. Once the tube is in place, the patient is asked to swallow. This device then measures the pressure and coordination of the muscle contractions and the pressure of the upper and lower esophageal sphincters. Abnormal esophageal contractions and a lax lower esophageal sphincter may be important contributing factors to GERD as well as esophageal motility disorders.

Additional testing that may be used include salivary pepsin testing, Heidelberg testing, the gastric emptying study and Xray.

SALIVARY PEPSIN TESTING

If reflux is occuring, pepsin may be detected in the saliva.

Non-invasive salivary pepsin testing may predict whether GERD, especially LPR is present. Pepsin is a protein digesting enzyme produced in the chief cells of the stomach. If reflux through the lower and upper esophageal sphincters is occurring, salivary pepsin can be present in the throat and be detected by this simple, non-invasive test. It is uncommon for clinics to offer this form of testing because the accuracy is in question, but it can be ordered directly by the patient on a website—pepsincheck.com

HEIDELBERG TESTING

Few offices perform the Heidelberg test, but I find it invaluable to determine whether the gastric parietal cells are making to much or too little acid.

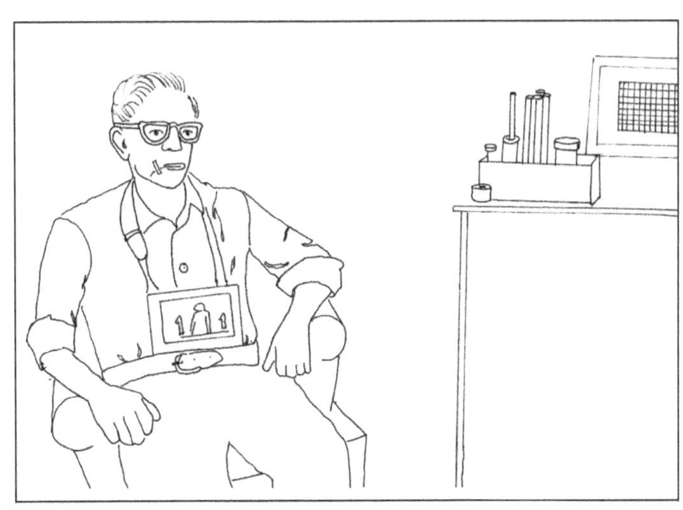

Fig. 4.6. Heidelberg pH capsule testing.

Unlike the BRAVO and pH impedance test procedures which measure esophageal pH, the Heidelberg test directly measures the acidity of a patient's stomach. The stomach may produce too much or too little acid, either of which can lead to symptoms and adverse health effects. Few offices perform this test, but I find the results informative and value having it available in my office. To find out where this test is available, go to www.phcapsule.com.

Procedure: The test involves swallowing a capsule, about the size of a standard vitamin pill, which is attached to a thin thread. The upper end of the thread is taped to the skin of the patient's cheek. Contained inside the capsule is a transmitter. The capsule enters the esophagus and then the stomach, where it measures the pH. The device tracks the acid level in the stomach as the patient swallows small amounts of a bicarbonate solution, neutralizing the hydrochloric acid. The acid level should gradually return to normal. The amount of time it takes for reacidification will point to hypochlorhydria, euchlorhydria, or hyperchlorhydria. After measurements have been taken, the capsule can then be removed through the mouth. This procedure is usually done in a seated position in an office rather than in an endoscopy suite, is well tolerated, and does not require sedation. The time required varies, but it generally takes about 2 hours.

GASTRIC EMPTYING STUDY (GES)

Considered the gold standard, the GES is the most specific test for diagnosing the speed at which the stomach empties.

Procedure: After eating a **radiolabelled** test meal, the amount of residual food in the stomach is measured hourly for four hours using a gamma camera. Some imaging centers will discontinue the test after two hours, but there is evidence that continuing the test for a period of four hours provides a higher sensitivity for detection of abnormal emptying.

The standardized meal contains a measured dose of radiolabelled tracer (99mTc-sulfur colloid) scrambled with 120 grams of liquid egg whites (Egg Beaters or generic), two slices of white toast, and 30 grams of strawberry jelly. It is all washed down with 120 mL of water.

Table 4.3. NORMAL GASTRIC EMPTYING TIMES
One hour: 30% to 90% meal retention
Two hours: Less than or equal to 60% meal retention
Four hours: Less than or equal to 10% meal retention
A retained meal value greater than 60% at two hours or 10% at four hours supports delayed gastric emptying
A retained meal value less than 70% at 30 minutes or less than 30% at one hour suggests rapid gastric emptying
Source: Seok JW, 2011

Patients who are vegan or gluten intolerant may be offered alternative test meals. A savory cake has been studied for this purpose in India (Somasundaram VH, 2014).

X-RAY/FLUOROSCOPY FILMS

An **esophagram** provides a moving x-ray picture of the esophagus during swallowing. It can show motility disorders as well as abnormal thickening. It can also reveal the presence of a hiatal hernia.

A full **upper GI series** (also called a barium swallow) reveals the esophagus, stomach, and duodenum.

Both the esophagram and the upper GI series involve swallowing barium, a white liquid contrast agent, which allows a radiologist to visualize the upper GI system under fluoroscopy. Unlike an upper endoscopy, x-rays cannot fully picture the tissue lining the esophagus, so it will not show some forms of inflammation or Barrett's esophagus. In addition, neither a normal upper endoscopy, nor a barium swallow exam rules out the diagnosis of GERD.

A full upper GI series has become less frequently used while endoscopy has become more common.

NON-STANDARD HOME TESTING

These are tests that I do not use, because there is no published research on them. I have included them because people frequently ask about them. I do not recommend relying on these.

Baking soda test—mix ¼ teaspoon baking soda in 4 ounces of water and drink before breakfast. It is considered normal to belch within 3 minutes of drinking the bicarbonate water. If it takes longer to belch, based on this empirical test, it is considered a suggestion of decreased stomach acid.

Lemon water test—proponents of this test suggest drinking juice made from ½ of a lemon mixed with water after eating a meal containing protein. Those who use this test consider an increase in heartburn an indication of excessive stomach acid and improvement in heartburn an indication of reduced stomach acid.

Betaine hydrochloride titration—proponents suggest taking betaine hydrochloride/pepsin capsules with meals containing protein to check for low stomach acid. At successive protein containing meals, an additional capsule is added up to a maximum of 1800 mg. If burning occurs at any stage, the suggestion is to cut down on the dosage or discontinue taking the capsules. If there is improvement in heartburn, this treatment may be continued.

CITATIONS

Koyyada A. Long-term use of proton pump inhibitors as a risk factor for various adverse manifestations. Therapie. 2021 Jan-Feb; 76(1):13-21. PMID: 32718584

Liu J, Li X, Fan L, Yang J et al. Proton pump inhibitors therapy and risk of bone diseases: An update meta-analysis. Life Sci. 2019 Feb 1; 218:213-223. PMID: 30605646

Fashner J, Gitu AC. Common gastrointestinal symptoms: risks of long-term proton pump inhibitor therapy. FP Essent. 2013 Oct; 413:29-39. PMID: 24124705

Erdogen A, Rao SSC. Small intestinal fungal overgrowth. Curr Gastroenterol Rep. 2015 Apr;17(4):16. PMID: 25786900

Arriola V, Tischendorf J, Musuuza J, Barker A et al. Assessing the Risk of Hospital-Acquired Clostridium Difficile Infection With Proton Pump Inhibitor Use: A Meta-Analysis , Infect Control Hosp Epidemiol. 2016 Dec; 37(12):1408-1417. PMID: 27677811

Lambert AA, Lam JO, Paik JJ, Ugarte-Gil C et al. Risk of community-acquired pneumonia with outpatient proton-pump inhibitor therapy: a systematic review and meta-analysis. PLoS One. 2015 Jun 4;10(6):e0128004. PMID: 26042842

Wei X, Yu J, Xu Z, Wang C, Wu Y. Incidence, Pathogenesis, and Management of Proton Pump Inhibitor-Induced Nephrotoxicity. Drug Saf. 2022 Jul; 45(7):703-712. PMID: 35641849

Vengrus CS, Delfino VD, Bignardi PR. Proton pump inhibitors use and risk of chronic kidney disease and end-stage renal disease. Minerva Urol Nephrol. 2021 Aug; 73(4):462-470. PMID: 33769018

Camilleri M, Donohoe K, Hasler WL, Lin HC, et al. Consensus recommendations for gastric emptying scintigraphy: a joint report of the American Neurogastroenterology and Motility Society and the Society of Nuclear Medicine. Am J Gastroenterol. 2008 Mar;103(3):753-63. PMID: 18028513

Seol JW, How to Interpret Gastric Emptying Scintigraphy. J Neurogastroenterol Motil. 2011 Apr; 17(2): 1890191. PMID: 21602998

Somasundaram VH, Subramanyam PS, Palaniswamy SS, A gluten-free vegan meal for gastric emptying scintigraphy: establishment of reference values and its utilization in the evaluation of diabetic gastroparesis Clin Nucl Med. 2014 Nov; 39(11):960-5. PMID: 25140554

FIVE

HOW STOMACH ACID IS PRODUCED AND SUPPRESSED

From the teeth onward down to the anus,
The GI tract sphincters are famous.
They keep every section,
In pH correction,
So digestive enzymes sustain us.

Glossary

adrenalin—a neurotransmitter in the sympathetic nervous system

acetylcholine—the major neurotransmitter in the parasympathetic nervous system

autonomic nervous system—the part of the nervous system responsible for unconscious control of the bodily functions, such as breathing, heartbeat, and digestive processes

cardiac sphincter—an alternate name for the lower esophageal sphincter because of its proximity to the heart

chief cell—the gastric cell that produces the enzyme called pepsin

epinephrine— another name for adrenalin

gastrin— a hormone which triggers proton pumps to make more acid

histamine—a proinflammatory substance produced by certain white blood cells and gut bacteria as well as cells in the body of the stomach

noradrenalin—a neurotransmitter similar to adrenalin

norepinephrine— another name for noradrenalin

neurotransmitter—a chemical needed to carry chemical impulses between adjacent nerves, thereby activating nerve transmission

parasympathetic nervous system— the rest and digest portion of the autonomic nervous system

parietal cell—a cell located in the gastric body, responsible for producing intrinsic factor and hydrochloric acid

pepsin— an enzyme that starts the process of digestion in the stomach

proton pump—a structure within parietal cells of the stomach that produces stomach acid

pylorus—the valve between the stomach and duodenum

sympathetic nervous system— the fight or flight activating portion of the autonomic nervous system

KEY QUESTIONS

What are the functional parts of the stomach?

By what processes is gastric acid produced and controlled?

How do acid suppressive treatments work?

How does the shape and physical structure of the stomach promote healthy function?

The stomach is a bag with a muscular drawstring at each end. It is divided into three main sections, each of which has specific functions and cell types.

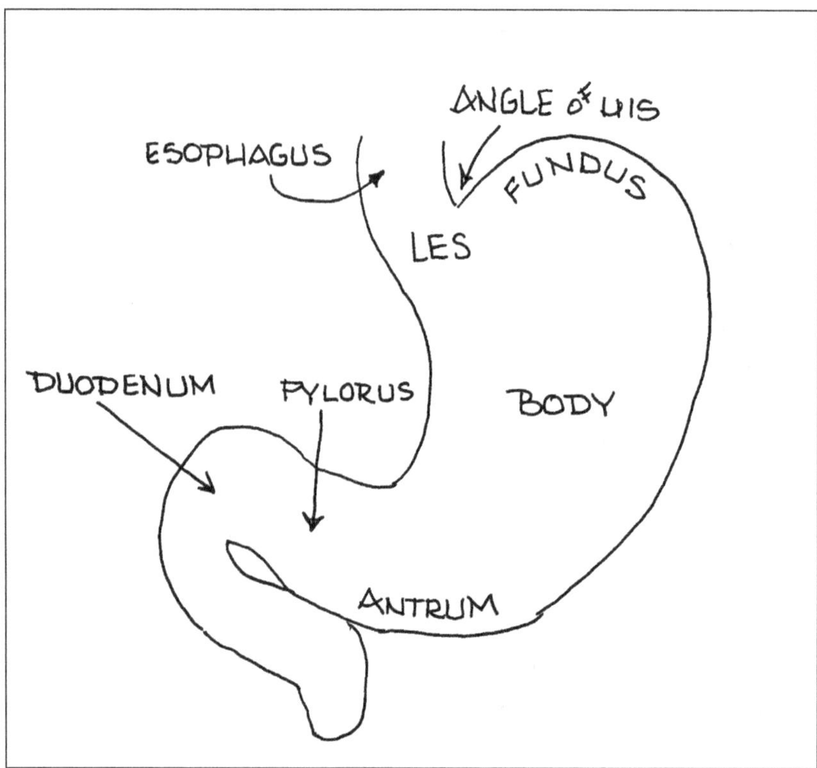

Fig. 5.1 Parts of the stomach.

The lower esophageal sphincter (LES), also known as the **cardiac sphincter**, is located at the bottom of the esophagus, where it meets the stomach.

Just below or alongside the LES is the fundus, the peninsular area that protrudes above the level of the LES. Just below is the main section of the stomach, referred to as the body of the stomach. The third section, located at the bottom of the bag is the **antrum.** At the end of the antrum is the **pylorus**, where the stomach meets the small intestines.

The entire stomach is lined with a mucus membrane made up of six types of cells: **epithelial cells**, **mucoid cells**, **chief cells**, **gastrin (G) cells**, **parietal cells**, and **endocrine cells**. Parietal cells, also referred to as oxyntic cells, are most predominant in the body of the stomach. Parietal cells are described as "pink, puffy, pillowy" cells where acid is produced in structures called proton pumps.

Parietal Cell Receptors

The parietal cell has the following 3 types of receptors or docking areas for specific chemicals that trigger the release of hydrochloric acid (HCl).

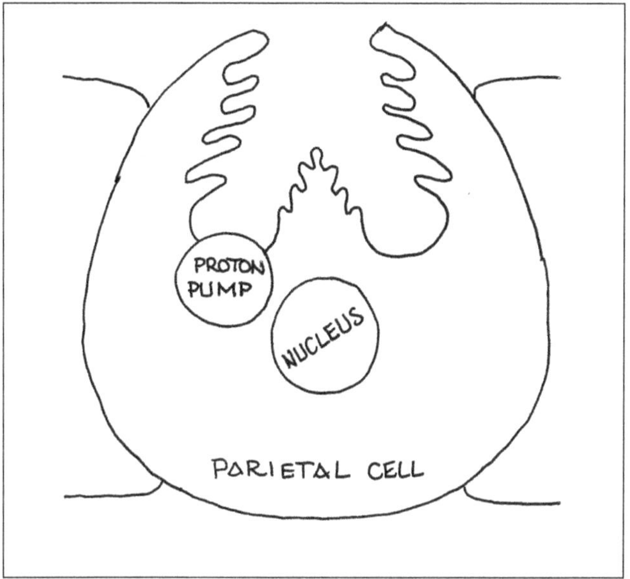

Fig. 5.2 Parietal cell with proton pump.

Histamine Receptor (H2 Receptor)

Histamine is an important chemical produced in several types of human cells including enterochromaffin-like cells (ECLs) which are scattered throughout the mucus membrane, and the mast cell which is a type of white blood cell. The histamine receptor's role in acid production was targeted by the earliest form of acid blocker—histamine-2 receptor antagonists (also called H2 blockers). Examples of this type of drug include cimetidine (Tagamet), ranitidine (Zantac), famotidine (Pepcid) and nizatidine (Axid).

Gastrin Receptor

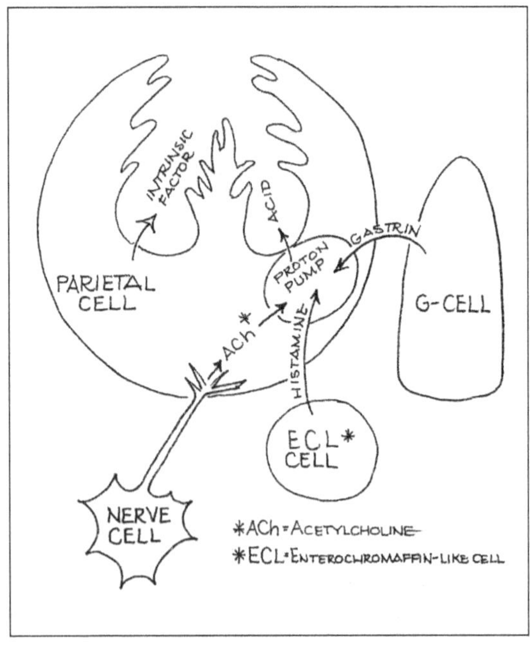

Fig. 5.3 Proton pump with its receptors.

Gastrin is a hormone made in G cells that are scattered throughout the mucosal lining of the antrum. Gastrin binds to the gastrin receptor, stimulating stomach acid production. Calcium salts can stimulate gastrin production. Milk protein and caffeine also stimulate gastrin. This may be the reason some people experience heartburn from consuming caffeine or dairy containing beverages. There is no heartburn medicine focused on blocking gastrin, but proton pump inhibitors and H2 receptor antagonists increase gastrin levels (Lee L, 2019 and McQuaid KR, 1991). Although gastrin levels are increased with these medicines, acidity does not increase because daily use of these medicines prevents the proton pump or histamine receptor from functioning.

Acetylcholine Receptor

Acetylcholine is one of the most important **neurotransmitters** in the gut. It activates the **parasympathetic nervous system**—the "rest and digest" part of the **autonomic nervous system**. The **vagus nerve** is the key parasympathetic nerve controlling multiple functions in the gut. It works in balance with the **sympathetic nervous system**—the "fight or flight" portion of the autonomic nervous system.

Case In Point: A child with severe heartburn which occurred nightly was brought to see me by her mother. It was found that the girl was eating rapidly so she could leave the table early and avoid being berated by her father. Bolting her food—coupled with anxiety—reduced parasympathetic and increased sympathetic activity, leading to heartburn.

Anticholinergic drugs such as dicyclomine (Bentyl) and diphenoxylate/atropine (Lomotil) target acetylcholine, but these drugs are prescribed to treat gut cramping and diarrhea, not specifically to block acid. Acid blocking can be a side effect. There is no acetylcholine receptor targeting drug that is prescribed for its direct effect on suppressing acid. There is no drug that addresses dysfunctional family interactions.

Acetylcholine is the neurotransmitter that activates the "rest and digest" (parasympathetic) portion of the autonomic nervous system.

The vagus nerve supplies parasympathetic nerve activity for the gut.

STRESS AND GASTRIC ACID SECRETION

Due to the complexity of the receptors in the parietal cell, emotional responses may either increase or decrease acid production. Some research indicates that the effect of emotion on acid secretion depends on personality. It may be that emotionally inhibited or repressed personality types tend to produce less acid when under stress, whereas extroverted people and those who easily express anger may produce more acid when under stress. Strong emotions affect acid secretion which may or may not affect reflux symptoms.

A BRIEF HISTORY OF HEARTBURN MEDICATIONS

The earliest heartburn medicines were called antacids. These were minerals such as sodium bicarbonate (baking soda), aluminum hydroxide (Gelusil), magnesium hydroxide (Milk of Magnesia) or calcium carbonate (Tums and Rolaids). Many products combine both aluminum and magnesium-based antacids (Maalox, Mylanta, etc). These minerals work by neutralizing acids. They do not act on the parietal cells where acid is produced, they simply neutralize the acid after it is secreted into the stomach. A serious concern regarding regular use of these antacids is excessive body storage of aluminum or calcium. Research suggests excessive aluminum has negative effects on the nervous system and, perhaps, also raises the risk of breast cancer (Pineau A, 2014 and Darbre PD, 2016). High concentrations of calcium in the body may lead to constipation, kidney stones and poor absorption of iron or zinc (Herzog P, 1982). More importantly, calcium salts stimulate gastrin leading to a vicious cycle of acid secretion. High levels of magnesium may cause diarrhea.

In the late 1970's the first H2 receptor antagonist became available. This type of acid blocker is discussed on page 65. Currently, the most common acid blockers bypass all the mechanisms discussed above and target the function of the entire proton pump. Examples of proton pump inhibitors include omeprazole (Prilosec), esomeprazole (Nexium), pantoprazole (Protonix), rabeprazole (Aciphex), lansoprazole (Prevacid) and dexlansoprazole (Dexilant). Some PPI products have an acid buffer added such as the combination of omeprazole plus sodium bicarbonate (Zegerid).

As of this writing, the newest acid blocker is Vonoprazan, which is in a class of medications called potassium-competitive acid blockers (PCAB) and is stronger at inhibiting acid than are the proton pump inhibitors. Vonoprazan is currently approved in the U.S. for use in treating *Helicobacter pylori* when combined with certain antibiotics (Kiyotoki S, 2020).

CITATIONS

Lee L, Ramos-Alvarez I, Ito T, Jensen RT, Insights into Effects/Risks of Chronic Hypergastrinemia and Lifelong PPI Treatment in Man Based on Studies of Patients with Zollinger-Ellison Syndrome. Int J Mol Sci. 2019 Oct 16;20(20):5128. PMID: 31623145

McQuaid KR, Much ado about gastrin. J Clin Gastroentero. 1991 Jun;13(3):249-54. PMID: 1676713

Pineau A, Faucommeau B, Sappino A-P, Deloncle R et al. If exposure to aluminium in antiperspirants presents health risks, its content should be reduced. J Trace Elem Med Biol. 2014 Apr;28(2):147-150. PMID: 24418462

Darbre PD. Aluminum and the human breast. Morphologie. 2016 Jun;100(329):65-74. PMID: 26997127

Herzog P, Holtermuller KH. Antacid therapy-changes in mineral metabolism. Scand J Gastroenterol Suppl. 1982;75:56-62. PMID: 6293043

Kiyotoki S, Nishikawa J, Sakaida I, Efficacy of Vonoprazan for Helicobacter pylori Eradication. Intern Med. 2020 Jan 15;59(2):153-161. PMID: 31243237

SIX

Melatonin—More Than Just a Sleep Hormone

Melatonin, as everyone knows,
Can help a person to doze,
It also prevents,
Mucosal events,
Of damage from acidic flows.

Glossary

archaea—a group of micro-organisms that are similar to, but evolutionarily distinct from bacteria

betaine—an amino acid with antioxidant and methyl donor functions. Sources include wheat bran, wheat germ, spinach, beets, and shrimp

circadian—biological functions that have a 24-hour cycle

cytokines—certain substances secreted by immune cells that either increase or decrease inflammation

enteroendocrine cells—cells in the digestive tract that produce hormones

free radical scavenger—a substance such as an antioxidant, that helps protect cells from tissue damage and genetic mutation

interleukin 1B—a pro-inflammatory cytokine

light pollution— brightening of the night sky caused by streetlights and other man-made sources, which has a disruptive effect on natural cycles

methionine—a sulfur containing amino acid that has antioxidant benefits

migrating motor complex—a nerve-muscle reflex triggered when the stomach is empty; it propels food and bacteria from the stomach to the ileocecal valve

nitric oxide—a neurotransmitter produced in white blood cells and other tissues; it relaxes arterial muscles and increases blood flow. It is derived from the amino acid arginine

placebo—the portion of a research study in which no treatment or a sham treatment is given to participants

portal vein—the vein which carries blood from the small intestine to the liver

prospective, randomized controlled trial is a form of research that is: **prospective**—starts with the present and follows participants forward in time, **randomized**—researchers decide randomly as to which participants in the trial receive the new treatment and which receive a placebo, or fake treatment, and **controlled**—the trial uses a control group for comparison. In the control group, the participants do not receive the new treatment but instead receive a placebo or reference treatment.

prostaglandins—a group of locally acting hormones involved in the regulation of inflammation, blood flow, blood clotting and the birth process

tryptophan—an amino acid precursor of serotonin and melatonin

tumor necrosis factor alpha—a pro-inflammatory chemical produced by certain white blood cells

KEY QUESTIONS

How does melatonin protect the esophagus from gastric acid?

What other important GI functions does melatonin control?

What is the GI clock and how may it become disrupted?

FUNCTIONS OF MELATONIN

Melatonin maintains the integrity of the esophagus and stomach through, in part, its control of GI mucosal blood flow. In a healthy body, melatonin is normally present in high amounts in the stomach, duodenum, and in the bile fluid. In fact, melatonin concentrations in the GI-mucosal lining have been measured at 100 – 400 times the level in the blood. Patients with upper digestive tract diseases such as erosive esophagitis and duodenal ulcer have reduced blood melatonin (Klupinska G, 2006).

Melatonin improves blood flow in the arteries supplying the digestive organs.

Melatonin may also protect the integrity of tight junctions between esophageal epithelial cells.

Melatonin improves blood flow in the arteries supplying the digestive organs. It regulates **nitric oxide** and **prostaglandins** which control the fine balance between pro-inflammatory and anti-inflammatory chemicals in the gut (Konturek SJ, 2007 and Majka J, 2018). Balanced levels of nitric oxide are also an important control over transient lower esophageal sphincter relaxations (TLESRs). As discussed in an earlier chapter, TLESRs may be a major cause of reflux when prolonged or frequent.

Animal studies have shown melatonin also protects the esophagus, stomach, and gallbladder from the damaging effects of acid, pepsin, and bile. It tends to reduce excessive gastric acid production thereby increasing levels of the GI hormone gastrin. Gastrin, in turn, increases the muscle tone of the lower esophageal sphincter, which may help to prevent reflux of gastric contents into the lower esophagus (Bang CS, 2019). Melatonin may also protect the integrity of tight junctions between esophageal epithelial cells, reducing the chance of dilated intercellular spaces associated with "leaky esophagus" (Tan J, 2014).

The countries with the highest known incidence of GERD are India, Greece, Romania, and Poland. A 2006 research team in Poland monitored melatonin levels through a 24-hour period in patients with upper digestive disorders and compared them to healthy controls. They found that the highest levels of melatonin were at 2 AM and those patients with non-erosive reflux had the highest levels of melatonin. Patients with erosive esophageal damage had much lower melatonin blood levels, while those with duodenal ulcers had the lowest of all (Klupinska G et al, 2006). These findings suggest that patients with the least tissue damage have the highest levels of melatonin which promotes GI mucosal healing and repair. It also lowers the levels of proinflammatory **cytokines interleukin 1B (IL-1B)** and **tumor necrosis factor alpha (TNF-alpha)** (Majka J, 2018). The amino acid **tryptophan**, found in turkey and other protein foods, is converted into serotonin, from which melatonin is derived. This conversion to melatonin occurs in the pineal gland and in the digestive tract.

In the GI tract, melatonin production is controlled by cycles of eating and fasting. In animal studies, meals containing tryptophan-rich foods significantly increased melatonin levels in the blood and digestive tract (Konturek SJ, 2007). Melatonin leaves the gut via the **portal vein** which carries it directly to the liver. After meals, the melatonin level in the portal vein is much higher than in the general circulation. Consuming the amino acid tryptophan can raise pineal production of melatonin six-fold and GI production ten-fold (Brzozowska I, 2014).

Studies of rats have shown oral doses of melatonin lead to the hormone being concentrated in the esophagus. Rats subjected to dripping of an acid-pepsin-bile solution into the esophagus for 2 hours a day developed erosions and even severe ulceration of the esophagus. When rats were given melatonin prior to the same challenge, mucosal lesions did not occur, suggesting a strong esophageal protective action (Konturek SJ, 2007).

A **prospective, randomized controlled trial** of a supplement containing melatonin, L-tryptophan, vitamin B6, folic acid, vitamin B12, **methionine** and **betaine** (not betaine hydrochloride) was conducted to evaluate its efficacy in treating patients with GERD. L-tryptophan was part of this supplement because, as mentioned above, an oral dose of L-tryptophan raises melatonin levels in the GI-tract and the liver by about ten-fold. Instead of comparing this experimental supplement to a **placebo**, the combination of melatonin with amino acids and vitamins was compared with a standard 20 mg daily dose of omeprazole, a commonly used proton pump inhibitor. Of the melatonin supplement group, 100% reported resolution of reflux symptoms after 40 days of treatment. Only 66% of the omeprazole group saw improvement in reflux (Pereira R de S, 2006). This research strongly suggests that melatonin may reduce the symptoms of GERD.

Melatonin helps protect from both internal and external irritants.

Several studies have proven no serious negative effects from oral melatonin even in large doses (Acuna-Castroviejo D, 2014). Based on its demonstrated safety, and the existing research pointing to protection and healing of the esophagus and the upper digestive tract in general, the use of melatonin supplementation appears to provide a protective effect against GERD.

The cells lining the upper GI tract are constantly battling internally produced corrosive substances such as acid and pepsin, as well as external factors introduced into the body, such as alcohol and drugs. Melatonin helps protect from both internal and external irritants.

THE GI CLOCK

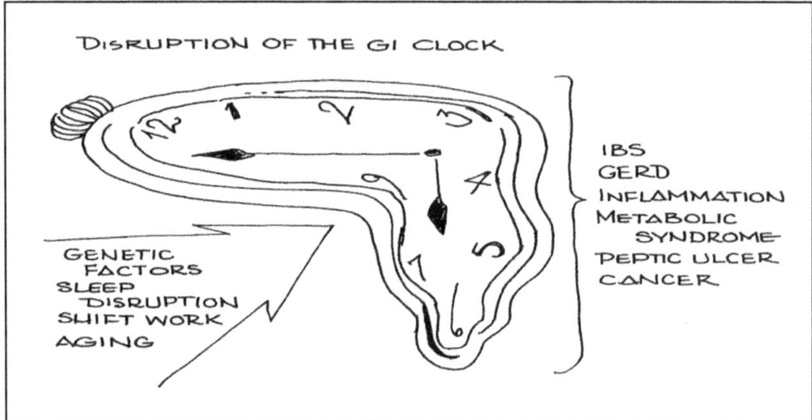

Fig. 6.1. The GI clock, with apologies to Salvador Dali. Concept from Konturek PC, 2011.

The daily rhythm of melatonin production in the brain by the pineal gland is controlled by cycles of exposure to light and dark.

This mechanism is why we think about sleep when we think about melatonin. Melatonin has major control over **circadian** and seasonal rhythms for most living organisms. The effect of light on the pineal gland is crucial to establishing rhythms of waking and sleeping. This gland is also sensitive to eating and fasting and plays an important role in the internal "GI clock". This clock controls cell function and repair and most aspects of the digestive process, including muscle activity and the secretion of hormones, acid, bicarbonate, and enzymes. The **migrating motor complex**, the cleansing wave of the small intestine, is just such a function of the GI clock. This wave is activated only when the stomach is empty, about four to five hours after meals. It propels food, bacteria, and debris along the entire eighteen-to-twenty foot length of the small intestine.

Many factors can decrease the effectiveness of the migrating motor complex, leading to overgrowth of bacteria, **archaea**, or yeast in the upper gut. The terms for such excess are small intestine bacterial overgrowth (SIBO), intestinal methanogen overgrowth (IMO) and small intestine fungal overgrowth (SIFO). Imbalanced normal flora are the major causes of irritable bowel syndrome and frequent contributing factors in GERD.

According to a 2011 article by Konturek PC and associates, modern life with its light pollution, 24-hour active city life, computer use, and phone screens, can lead to disruption of the body clock, creating serious digestive problems (Konturek PC, 2011).

Disruption of circadian physiology, due to sleep disturbance or shift work, may result in various gastrointestinal diseases, such as IBS, GERD, or peptic ulcer disease.

CITATIONS

Klupinska G.A., Wisniowska-Jarosinska M., Harsiuk A., Chojnacki C., Stec-Michska K., Błasiak J., Reiter R.J., Chojnacki J. Nocturnal secretion of melatonin in patients with upper digestive tract disorders. J. Physiol. Pharmacol. 2006;57:41–50. PMID: 17218759

Konturek S.J., et al. Protective influence of melatonin against acute esophageal lesions involves prostaglandins, nitric oxide and sensory nerves. J. Physiol. Pharmacol. 2007;58:371–387. PMID: 17622703

Majka J et al, Melatonin in Prevention of the Sequence from Reflux Esophagitis to Barrett's Esophagus and Esophageal Adenocarcinoma: Experimental and Clinical Perspectives. Int J Mol Sci. 2018 Jul; 19(7): 2033. PMID: 30011784

Bang SB, Yang YJ, Baik GH. Melatonin for the treatment of gastro- esophageal reflux disease; protocol for a systematic review and meta-analysis. Medicine (Baltimore). 2019 Jan; 98(4): e14241. PMID: 30681611

Tan J, Wang Y, Xia Y, Zhang N et al. Melatonin protects the esophageal epithelial barrier by suppressing the transcription, expression and activity of myosin light chain kinase through ERK1/2 signal transduction. Cell Physiol Biochem. 2014;34(6):2117-27. PMID: 25562159

Brzozowska I, Strzalka M,Drozdowicz D, Konturek SJ, et al. Mechanisms of esophageal protection, gastroprotection and ulcer healing by melatonin. implications for the therapeutic use of melatonin in gastroesophageal reflux disease (GERD) and peptic ulcer disease. Curr Pharm Des. 2014;20(30):4807-15. PMID: 24251671

Pereira R de S et al, Regression of gastroesophageal reflux disease symptoms using dietary supplementation with melatonin, vitamins and aminoacids: comparison with omeprazole. J Pineal Res . 2006 Oct;41(3):195-200. PMID 16948779

Acuna-Castroviejo D., Escames G., Venegas C., Díaz-Casado M.E., Lima-Cabello E., López L.C., Rosales-Corral S., Tan D.X., Reiter R.J. Extrapineal melatonin: Sources, regulation, and potential functions. Cell. Mol. Life Sci. 2014;71:2997–3025. PMID: 24554058

Konturek PC, Brzozwska T, Konturek SJ. Gut clock: implication of circadian rhythms in the gastrointestinal tract. J Physiol Pharmacol. 2011 Apr;62(2):139-50. PMID: 21673361

SEVEN

What Determines Whether Reflux Leads to Esophagitis?

NERD is a comical name
For erosion-free refluxive fame.
What leads into GERD,
Instead of just NERD?
This chapter is here to explain.

Glossary

Barrett's esophagus—changes in the cell lining of the lower esophagus, from stratified squamous to columnar; occurring in some patients with chronic gastroesophageal reflux.

columnar cells—taller than they are wide, these are typical cells found in the stomach, small intestine, and large intestine

dilated intercellular spaces—widening of the microscopic space between mucosal lining cells of the esophagus

functional dyspepsia—recurring indigestion with no diagnosis explaining the symptoms

metaplastic cells—a change in cell structure to a form that is not normally found in that area of the body

paracellular—the space between cells that line the mucous membrane

stem cells—primitive cells from which all other cells with specialized functions are generated

KEY QUESTIONS

Can the esophagus remain undamaged despite having GERD?

What is meant by visceral hypersensitivity, sustained esophageal contractions and abnormal tissue resistance?

What are the factors other than acid that can damage the esophagus?

Much of the confusion in reflux stems from the fact that heartburn and other reflux symptoms can be caused by many things, with only one of them being acid reflux. If the "diagnosis" of GERD is made with a hunch and a PPI challenge or just a questionnaire, the diagnosis is wrong up to 37% of the time. If a gastroenterologist, rather than a family practice physician, makes the diagnosis, the accuracy improves by only 7%. According to John Dent writing in the journal GUT, "[*using*] *the symptom-based diagnosis of GERD by the Reflux Disease Questionnaire, family practitioners and gastroenterologists had moderate and similar accuracy. Symptom response to a two-week course of 40 mg of esomeprazole (Nexium—a PPI) did not increase the diagnostic accuracy* (Dent J, 2010)." Guidelines suggest that PPIs should be taken 30-60 minutes before a meal for best response (Katz PO et al, 2022).

When a patient does not respond to the trial of PPI, the next steps should be some form of diagnostic testing, as described in chapter four.

When an upper endoscopy shows a normal appearing esophagus, but the person has heartburn, one must consider the following mechanism: When the esophagus is exposed to repeated reflux, the microscopic spaces between the cells that line the lower esophagus enlarge. These **dilated intercellular spaces** (DIS) occur in both nonerosive (NERD) and erosive reflux disease. These structural changes result in an increase in permeability between the cells (**paracellular**), allowing refluxed fluid to reach and stimulate chemical pain receptors in nerve endings deep to the esophageal lining cells. This stimulation sends a message to the brain which triggers pain perception (Barlow WJ, 2005).

Dilated intercellular spaces are not found by an upper endoscopy exam, nor by typical biopsy of esophageal tissue. DIS is found only when biopsy specimens are examined with an electron microscope which is mainly used in research. In 2001, Villanacci V et al. devised a computer assisted method that can be used to allow standard light-microscopy techniques to see DIS. Having read many hundreds of esophageal biopsy reports, I have not seen this used or reported. Since virtually all people with the various types of reflux, and 30% of people without reflux, have DIS, we can almost assume it is present. There is a strong correlation between the duration of esophageal acid exposure and DIS.

Two Main Categories of Reflux (Plus a Third)

The effects of esophageal reflux on the esophageal lining can be divided into two main types—erosive esophagitis (EE) and non-erosive reflux disease (NERD). Up to 70% of people with frequent prolonged gastric reflux manage to avoid having swelling, visible irritation, or erosions in the esophagus (Zentilin P, 2017).

Acid reflux stems is only one possible cause of heartburn.

If GERD is investigated merely by a PPI trial, the diagnosis is wrong 30–37% of the time.

A third category is **Barrett's esophagus**. Here chronic reflux stimulates **stem cells** to shift from transitioning into the typical squamous type of esophageal lining cell and instead change into **metaplastic cells** (similar to intestinal cells). In cases where there is more than a 3-centimeter area of Barrett's metaplasia, a tiny fraction of patients can develop a type of cancer called esophageal adenocarcinoma. It is believed that EE is most likely to turn into Barrett's and that NERD rarely does (Hershcovici T, 2010). Both EE and Barrett's can be treated and shifted back to normal esophageal tissue (Caygill CPJ, 2011).

Erosive esophagitis and NERD are very different conditions. The duration of esophageal acid exposure correlates with severity of erosive esophagitis (EE). Esophageal exposure to acid and pepsin is increased in more severe reflux. Despite this, research does not support a significant difference in the amount of acid secreted by the stomach of patients with NERD or EE, but an increasing number of reflux events per day and a longer duration of the esophageal exposure to the acid are found in EE and even more so in Barrett's (Hershcovici T, 2010). Although acid reflux gives rise to similar symptoms with or without erosion, the mechanism of acid injury may be different.

THREE MECHANISMS MAY EXPLAIN THE SENSATION OF HEARTBURN IN NERD PATIENTS

ESOPHAGEAL VISCERAL HYPERSENSITIVITY

NERD heartburn may be related to a heightened perception of distention or muscular contractions of the esophagus. I often explain this phenomenon as someone who perceives the normally imperceptible muscle contractions differently than most people. For those with hypersensitivity, the passage of food or fluid in the digestive tract is experienced as pain or burning. Miwa and colleagues found that NERD patients had lower pain thresholds when either acid or salt water was infused into the esophagus. This was true when comparing them to normal controls as well as people diagnosed with erosive esophagitis and Barrett's esophagus (Miwa H, 2004 and Nagahara A, 2006).

A study by Noh et al. showed that NERD is found more often in the same patients that have functional bowel disorders. These include GI conditions such as irritable bowel syndrome (IBS) and **functional dyspepsia**. This overlap in digestive conditions is less common in EE patients. The study clearly demonstrated that having NERD increases a patient's risk of having IBS. GERD patients who also suffer from IBS are less likely to respond to standard acid suppression treatment as compared to those without a functional bowel disorder.

NERD patients have exceptionally high levels of melatonin.

Sustained Esophageal Contractions

There is evidence that some people have more intense or longer lasting esophageal muscle contractions which can be perceived as burning or pressure. I have not found any well-founded theories explaining the causes of these prolonged contractions.

Abnormal Tissue Resistance

Proposed causes for abnormal tissue resistance include cigarette smoking, dehydration, impaired saliva production, nutritional factors, etc.

As discussed in chapter six, research has shown that patients with reflux, but no damage to the esophagus (NERD) have higher levels of protection from inflammation because of exceptionally high upper GI tract levels of melatonin. Those with damage from reflux have lower levels, and those with ulcers (the deepest damage) have the lowest level of the hormone (Klupinska G et al, 2006).

Additionally, there is early evidence that the state of the bacteria living in the upper digestive tract play a role in whether esophagitis occurs (Giovanni B et al, 2019). Drug therapy to eradicate *Helicobacter pylori* (which lives in the stomach) has been proven to *increase* the risk of developing reflux esophagitis. This effect is true whether, or not, patients have had esophagitis prior to the eradication therapy, and there is no improvement in reflux-related symptoms with *H. pylori* treatment (Sugimoto M et al, 2020). It is important to know that the standard dictum for *H. pylori* is "Test and Treat". This means that if you test positive for *H. pylori* bacteria, you will be treated for it—even if the condition you have is not caused by the bacteria. In this situation, if you have reflux, your symptoms may not improve after this treatment. I discuss this in more detail in chapter thirteen.

Killing Helicobacter pylori bacteria increases the risk of developing erosive esophagitis.

CITATIONS

Dent J et al, Accuracy of the diagnosis of GORD by questionnaire, physicians and a trial of proton pump inhibitor treatment: the Diamond Study. Gut. 2010 Jun;59(6):714-21. PMID: 20551454

Katz PO, Dunbar KB, Schnoll-Sussman FH, Greer KB et al. ACG Clinical Guideline for the Diagnosis and Management of Gastroesophageal Reflux Disease The American Journal of Gastroenterology: January 2022 - Volume 117 - Issue 1 - p 27-56. PMID: 34807007

Barlow WJ, Orlando RC. The pathogenesis of heartburn in non-erosive reflux disease: a unifying hypothesis. Gastroenterology. 2005;128:771–778. PMID: 15765412

Villanacci V et al, Dilated intercellular spaces as markers of reflux disease: histology, semiquantitative score and morphometry upon light microscopy. Digestion. 2001;64(1):1-8. PMID: 11549831

Zentilin P et al, Complexity and diversity of gastroesophageal reflux disease phenotypes. Minerva Gastroenterol Dietol. 2017 Sep;63(3):198-204. PMID: 28272380

Hershcovici T, Fass R, Nonerosive Reflux Disease (NERD) - An Update. J Neurogastroenterol Motil. 2010 Jan; 16(1): 8–21. PMID: 20535321

Miwa H, Minoo T, Hojo M, et al. Oesophageal hypersensitivity in Japanese patients with non-erosive gastro-oesophageal reflux diseases. Aliment Pharmacol Ther. 2004;20(suppl 1):112–117. PMID: 15298616

Nagahara A, Miwa H, Minoo T, et al. Increased esophageal sensitivity to acid and saline in patients with nonerosive gastro-esophageal reflux disease. J Clin Gastroenterol. 2006;40:891–895. PMID: 17063106

Klupinska G.A., Wisniowska-Jarosinska M., Harsiuk A., Chojnacki C., et al. Nocturnal secretion of melatonin in patients with upper digestive tract disorders. J. Physiol. Pharmacol. 2006;57:41–50. PMID: 17218759

Noh YW et al, Overlap of Erosive and Non-erosive Reflux Diseases With Functional Gastrointestinal Disorders According to Rome III Criteria. J Neurogastroenterol Motil. 2010 Apr; 16(2): 148–156. PMID: 20535345

Caygill CPJ et al, Barrett's esophagus: surveillance and reversal. Ann N Y Acad Sci. 2011 Sep;1232:196-209. PMID: 21950814

Giovanni B et al, Proton pump inhibitors and dysbiosis: Current knowledge and aspects to be clarified. World J Gastroenterol 2019 Jun 14; 25(22): 2706–2719. PMID: 31235994

Sugimoto M et al, Endoscopic Reflux Esophagitis and Reflux-Related Symptoms after Helicobacter pylori Eradication Therapy: Meta-Analysis. J Clin Med. 2020 Sep; 9(9): 3007. PMID: 32961949

EIGHT

How Lifestyle Factors Affect GERD

"Reduce CARBS" is something we've heard,
These common admonishing words,
From Paleo to Keto,
This mnemonic that we know
Reminds us of what causes GERD.

Glossary

body composition analysis—a measurement of body percentages of fat, water and muscle

body mass index (BMI)—a ratio calculated by dividing one's weight in kilograms by the square of one's height in meters. This is used as an indicator of obesity, overweight, normal weight and underweight status

central adiposity/apple fat—the fat that surrounds the abdominal internal organs measured by waist circumference

crossover trial—a type of clinical trial in which all participants receive the same two or more treatments, but the order in which they receive them depends on the group to which they are randomly assigned

DeMeester score—a composite score of the esophageal acid exposure during pH monitoring tests. It has been used to definitively diagnose GERD since the 1970s

gluteofemoral adiposity/pear fat— the type of fat measured by thigh circumference, hip circumference, and fat deposits on the legs

glycemic load—how specific foods affect blood sugar levels

meta-analysis—the statistical analysis of data from several independent studies of the same topic, in order to summarize overall trends

nonsteroidal anti-inflammatory drugs—a class of drugs which reduce pain, decrease inflammation, decrease fever, and reduce the formation of blood clots (eg. Ibuprofen, aspirin, naproxen)

prospective trial—a study that observes a group of people over a period of time to gather information and record outcomes

supine— lying face upward, on the back

systematic review— a compilation of research used to answer a specific question. It is done by collecting and summarizing all research evidence that fits pre-specified eligibility criteria

KEY QUESTIONS

How may I alter my diet and lifestyle to reduce heartburn and reflux?

What does scientific research say about these modifications?

Below is a mnemonic device to list the more important lifestyle factors that can trigger or increase heartburn and other reflux symptoms. It is unlikely that they are all significant triggers for any one person, but one or more may be important. People with reflux may choose to avoid these foods, drinks, drugs (check with your doctor before making any changes to your prescription medications) or activities. This can be done one factor at a time based on individual diet and lifestyle. This may help to narrow down just what impact each one has on an individual's symptoms.

A "Reduce **CARBS,** Relieve Reflux" Mnemonic

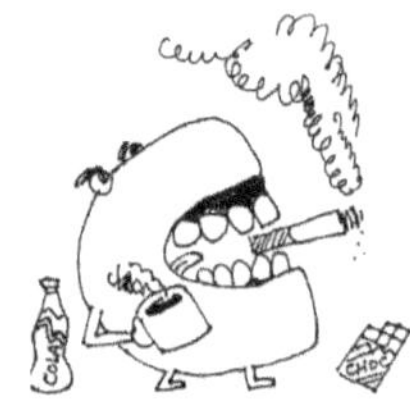

Cola (soda in general), coffee, chocolate, cigarettes (tobacco in general)

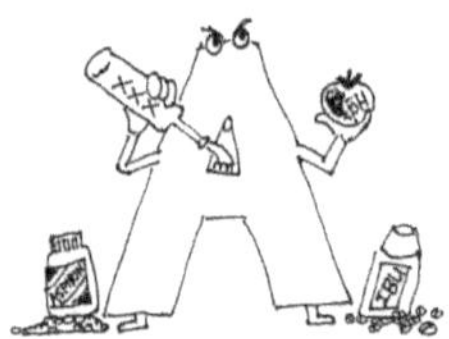

Alcohol, acidic foods, aspirin (and other over the counter pain and inflammation medicines)

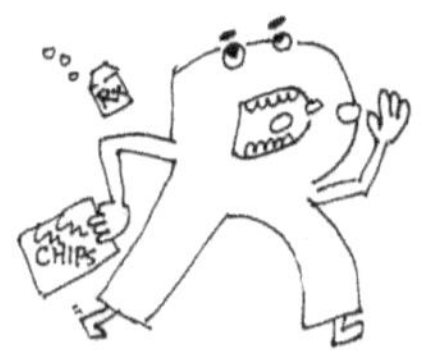

Refined carbohydrates (excess carbohydrate intake including unrefined such whole grains or starchy vegetables—see chapter nine); rapid eating; Rx (certain prescription medicines discussed in chapter one)

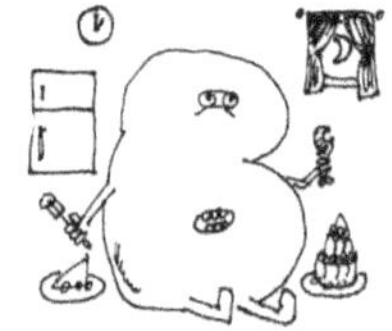

Breathing shallowly, big meals (eating too much at a meal); big waist circumference; bedtime eating or eating within 3 hours of going to bed

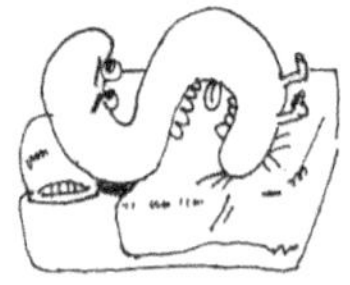

Saturated fat, (high intake of any type of fat); spicy food; sensitivity to specific foods; snacking; sleeping position

The following is the mnemonic in more detail:

COLA AND OTHER SODA

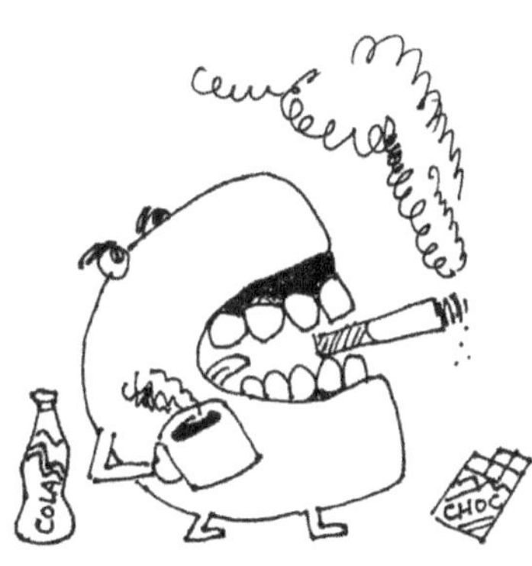

Consuming carbonated soft drinks causes almost immediate acid pH in the lower esophagus.

There are commercial acid-free coffees that taste like regular coffee, which theoretically may be less likely to trigger GERD or esophagitis.

The Melbourne Collaborative Cohort Study is a large **prospective trial** which found that carbonated beverages increased the risk of GERD in both men and women (Wang SE, 2021). Agrawal A, 2005 found that carbonated soft drinks were highly acidic and caused almost immediate acid pH in the lower esophagus. Another study found that although extreme acidity lasted only 90 seconds, an acid pH of less than 4.0 could persist for up to 13 minutes after exposure (Shoenut JP, 1998). Others speculate that carbonated drinks cause more distention of the stomach, increasing intragastric pressure which may cause laxity of the LES. Perhaps the best evidence of a mechanism of carbonated beverages causing reflux comes from Pouderoux et al. Their research found that carbonated rather than distilled water increased the retention of food and liquid in the gastric fundus, putting stomach contents and increased pressure where it would have the most reflux potential.

COFFEE

Drinking espresso, filtered coffee or instant coffee significantly raises serum gastrin levels within 15 minutes of consumption. This effect on gastrin, a potent stimulator of acid production by the parietal cells in the body of the stomach, wears off after about an hour (Papakonstantino E, 2016). A **meta-analysis** of 15 studies did not find that the symptom of heartburn correlated with coffee consumption, but the presence of erosive esophagitis on upper endoscopy, did (Kim J, 2014). There are commercial acid-free coffees that taste like regular coffee, which theoretically may be less likely to trigger GERD or esophagitis.

CHOCOLATE

According to Surdea-Blaga et al, chocolate induces reflux and increases the lower esophageal exposure to acid. Research published at Stanford University adds that chocolate reduces lower esophageal sphincter pressure (Kaltenbach, 2006).

CIGARETTES

A meta-analysis of smoking as a risk of Barrett's esophagus found a consistent association. The greater number of packs per day over years of smoking increased the risk (Andrici J, 2013). In smokers, laryngopharyngeal reflux symptoms and upper endoscopy findings significantly improved after two months of tobacco cessation (Dinc ASC, 2020). Kahrilas reports that smokers have chronically diminished LES pressure and smoking increases the rate of reflux events. The most important mechanisms are thought to be decreased effectiveness of saliva in clearing refluxed material from the esophagus as well as increased intra-abdominal pressure.

Smokers have decreased LES pressure and more reflux events.

Alcohol

Alcohol consumption can reduce the LES pressure, which facilitates reflux. Alcohol also has a direct toxic effect on the esophageal mucosa, predisposing to acid/pepsin injury (Ness-Jensen E, 2017). German researchers report that alcohol use reduces the strength of contraction of the lower esophagus leading to decreased clearance of refluxed material (Franke A, 2005). These effects also increase the risk of esophageal cancer. A meta-analysis of twenty-nine research studies found that any regular use of alcohol increases the rate of reflux by just under 50% compared to non-drinkers or occasional drinkers. Alcohol use is more of a risk for erosive esophagitis rather than NERD (Pan J, 2019).

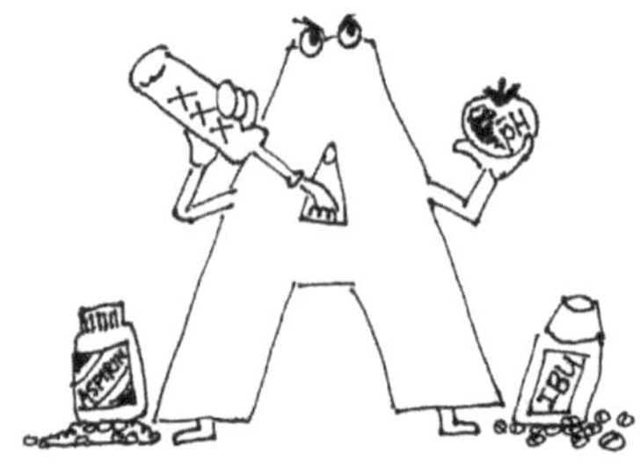

Alcohol also has a direct toxic effect on the esophageal mucosa, predisposing to acid/ pepsin injury.

Acidic Foods

The consumption of citrus fruit, vinegar and tomato can either aggravate or ameliorate GERD. I often ask my reflux patients how they respond if they take a teaspoon of apple cider vinegar in two ounces of water just before a meal. Some get relief and others feel more burning and reflux symptoms. My theory is that patients with erosive esophagitis or gastritis are more sensitive to the acidity of vinegar and feel it as burning or pain. In addition, I theorize that those with hypochlorhydria and NERD often respond positively to the addition of vinegar, lemon juice, bitter herbs or betaine hydrochloride capsules taken with meals. A 2018 Italian study found that daily intake of citrus fruit and tomato along with a sugar-free diet was effective in treating GERD. They suggest that the acids in lemon, orange and tomato lowered the pH of the stomach which reduced the production of gastrin and therefore hydrochloric acid, relieving heartburn symptoms (Langella C, 2018).

Consuming acidic foods may either increase or decrease reflux symptoms.

Aspirin and Non-steroidal Anti-inflammatory Drugs (NSAIDs)

A 2018 meta-analysis of ten research studies from around the world found a significant increase in reflux symptoms in people

Aspirin disrupts the normal cytoprotective barrier in the stomach and esophagus.

Nonsteroidal anti-inflammatory drugs should be prescribed with caution for people with GERD.

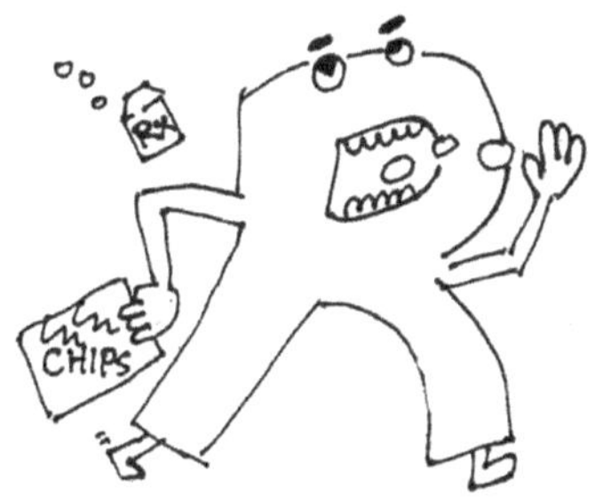

Women eating a lower carbohydrate diet had relief from GERD within ten weeks.

taking NSAIDs or aspirin (25.5%) compared to non-users (19.6%). These medications can also cause upper GI erosions and ulcerations. Aspirin is sold in both low dose (81 mg tablets) and regular dosage (325 or 500 mg tablets). A Japanese study of over 5500 people undergoing upper endoscopy compared subjects who took low dose aspirin compared to non-users. The incidence of erosive esophagitis was only 3% higher in the aspirin group, but there was a 10% higher risk for developing a peptic ulcer. According to Zographos et al, "aspirin disrupts the normal cytoprotective (cell protective) barrier in the mucosa of the stomach and a similar process has been found to occur in the esophagus… Esophageal emptying is slow in the elderly, resulting in a prolonged exposure of the mucosa to their irritant action. Nonsteroidal anti-inflammatory drugs should be prescribed with caution in the presence of symptomatic gastroesophageal reflux."

Refined and Excessive Dietary Carbohydrates

A very low carbohydrate diet may be effective for reflux (Surdea-Blaga T, 2019). It was found to be significantly effective in a study of eight obese subjects with GERD. 24-hour esophageal pH impedance testing was performed before and after a six-day diet containing less than 20 grams of carbohydrate per day. The DeMeester score (see Chapter four) for reflux dropped from an average of 34.7 to 14.0 (normal is less than 14.7). The percentage of time the esophageal pH was more acidic than 4.0 dropped by half (Austin GL, 2006). In another study, 33 obese white women and 9 obese black women followed a 16-week diet which was lower in simple and complex carbohydrate and higher in fat (saturated, polyunsaturated, and monounsaturated). The control group was 70 white women and 32 black women with comparable body types but no GERD symptoms (Pointer SD, 2017). Prior to the dietary intervention, the women with GERD had been eating a diet with a higher **glycemic load,** which included more total carbohydrate, sucrose, total sugar, and starch. They had higher insulin resistance and inflammation levels. Body composition analysis, blood inflammatory markers, glucose, and insulin as well as GERD symptoms and use of GERD medications were monitored during the study. The overwhelming result was that <u>all</u> the women with reflux had resolution of GERD symptoms within ten weeks and discontinued their reflux medications. The white women had the highest carbohydrate intakes before starting the study and had the greatest reduction in insulin resistance by following the

16-week low carbohydrate diet. All the women lost similar amounts of weight.

Certain indigestible forms of carbohydrate, such as psyllium seed powder or fenugreek fiber powder, may reduce reflux (DiSilvestro RA, 2011). A Russian study using a sucrose sweetened psyllium seed powder (five grams three times/day) found a significant increase in LES pressure and significant reduction in acidic and weakly acidic reflux episodes. Reflux time dropped in half (Morozov S, 2018). Some have suggested that the gel that forms when psyllium fiber is mixed with water may create a barrier which prevents reflux. It is interesting that fenugreek is also used in traditional medicine for insulin resistance since this is also a risk factor for GERD (Zhou C, 2020) .

Consuming psyllium seed powder significantly increased LES pressure and reduced acid reflux.

Rapid Eating

Increased numbers and duration of TLESRs are thought to be an important cause of GERD. TLESRs are triggered when the stomach is distended by solids, liquids and/or gas and the LES opens for longer periods of time than needed to allow food to pass. Remaining open permits the venting of pressure and gas. A study of 20 normal adults (13 women and 7 men without reflux) measured the difference in 24-hour pH impedance results between identical meals eaten either in five minutes or eaten in thirty minutes (Wilde SM, 2004). The two test meals were spaced a day apart. A significant increase in the number of reflux events followed the five-minute meal compared to the thirty minute meal. The increased reflux was predominantly non-acid in the first hour after eating and more acidic in the second hour. Of note: An earlier study showed that subjects with hiatal hernia had twice the number of TLESRs, so a combination of rapid eating, larger meals and a hiatal hernia may be the most significant trigger for reflux (Kahrilas PJ, 2000).

Eating a meal in five minutes increases reflux, compared to eating the same meal in thirty minutes.

Rx-prescription Medications Causing or Increasing GERD

Asthma Medications

albuterol (Ventolin, Proventil)

metaproterenol (Alupent)

pirbuterol (Maxair)

terbutaline (Brethaire)

isoetharine (Bronkosol)

levalbuterol (Xopenex)

salmeterol (Serevent).

HEART AND HYPERTENSION MEDICATIONS

isosorbide mononitrate (Imdur, Monoket)

isosorbide dinitrate (Isordil)

propranolol (Inderal)

amlodipine (Norvasc)

diltiazem (Cardizem)

felodipine (Plendil)

nicardipine (Cardene)

nifedipine (Adalat, Procardia)

OSTEOPOROSIS MEDICATIONS

bisphosphonates (Fosomax, Boniva and Actonel)

ADDITIONAL DRUGS

tricyclic antidepressants (used to treat irritable bowel syndrome)

   amitriptyline (Elavil)

   imipramine (Tofranil)

   desipramine (Norpramin)

   nortriptyline (Pamelor, Aventyl)

anticholinergics such as atropine in Lomotil

narcotics such as morphine, oxycodone, Vicodin, etc (sources differ on this effect)

benzodiazepine sedatives such as diazepam (Valium) and barbiturate sedatives

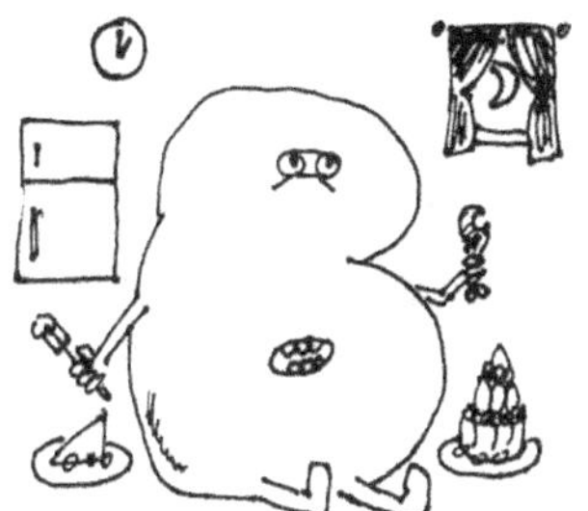

Diaphragmatic breathing reduces GERD symptoms and PPI use.

BREATHING SHALLOWLY

Eherer A, 2014 showed that training GERD patients to use diaphragmatic breathing can strengthen the LES. They conducted a randomized trial and used breathing exercises as the intervention. GERD patients using diaphragmatic breathing techniques were found to have fewer GERD symptoms as well as improved quality of life, better pH-impedance findings, and reduced PPI use.

BIG MEALS (OVEREATING)

Similar to rapid eating, large meals can distend the stomach enough to trigger more TLESRs and increase reflux symptoms.

Big Waist Circumference

Compared to lower weight adults, the odds of having GERD are three times greater in obese men and four times greater in obese women (Pointer SD, 2016). A study of 743 subjects in Taiwan found increasing waist circumference and **body mass index** (**BMI**) is associated with insulin resistance, rising blood sugar levels and GERD. These were most strongly associated in men (Hsu CS, 2011). Two meta-analyses found a positive association among increasing BMI, GERD symptoms and complications such as erosive esophagitis (Corley D, 2006 and Hampel H, 2005).

Bigger waist measurements increase GERD in men and women.

Of note, people with increased girth at the waist have more GERD than people whose extra weight is in the buttocks and legs. Singh et al found that **central adiposity** ("apple fat") leads to nearly twice the risk of developing GERD with erosive esophagitis than other body types (Singh S, 2013). In contrast, men with increased hip circumference or **gluteofemoral** ("pear-fat") girth were protected against developing GERD symptoms, erosive esophagitis, type 2 diabetes, cardiovascular disease as well as Barrett's esophagus (Rubenstein JH, 2013 and Kendall BJ, 2016). The protective effect was minimally present, but not significant for women.

Bedtime Meals

Eating within three hours of bedtime increases the risk of reflux by as much as seven-and-a-half times (Zhang M 2021).

Saturated Fat

It is often said that consuming saturated fat increases GERD. While some studies have shown that fat increases the perception of reflux and causes more symptoms in patients with gastroparesis (Homko CJ, 2015), a recent study of over 3000 Iranians using questionnaires to assess reflux and dietary fat, found no correlation (Ebrahimpour-Koujan S, 2021). Overall, research on dietary fat is less conclusive than research on carbohydrate intake and GERD.

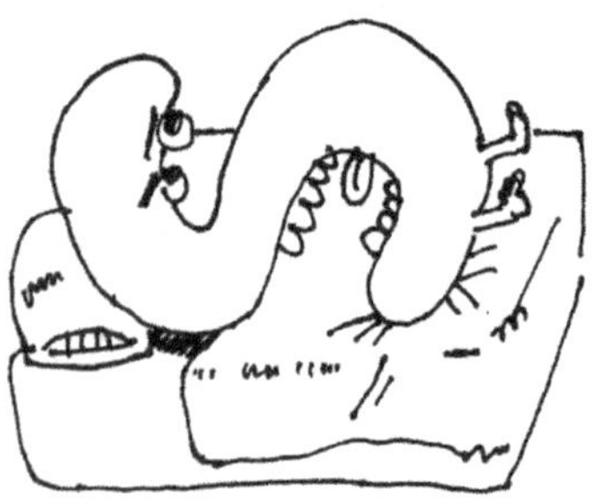

Spicy Food

There are many variables in researching the effect of spicy food on reflux symptoms because individuals respond uniquely to the wide variety of spices. An Iranian questionnaire and symptom study of over 4600 men and women found high consumption of spicy foods was associated with a greater risk of heartburn in men, but not in women. The men eating spicy food more than ten times per week had three times more heartburn than men who did not eat spicy food. Another study found that occasional ingestion of chili may aggravate abdominal pain and burning symptoms whereas frequent, long-term use of chili in food has been found to improve functional dyspepsia and GERD symptoms (Gonlachanvit S, 2010).

SENSITIVITY TO SPECIFIC FOODS

Published case studies have shown that individuals have resolved reflux by removing specific foods to which they are sensitive (Vora A, 2021).

SNACKING

A pilot study found that meal spacing for two weeks with no snacking resolved heartburn in 75% of subjects with erosive esophagitis. By eating two meals per day with only liquids between, the subjects were able to discontinue heartburn medication (Randhawa MA, 2015).

SLEEPING POSITION

During the daytime, the average person produces over a liter of saliva. About every minute, the saliva is swallowed, bathing the esophagus in mildly alkaline fluid. This can help neutralize refluxed material from the stomach. During sleep, we swallow less frequently, and secrete less saliva. Research shows that esophageal acid clearance is significantly slower during sleep, even in studies of people sleeping upright!

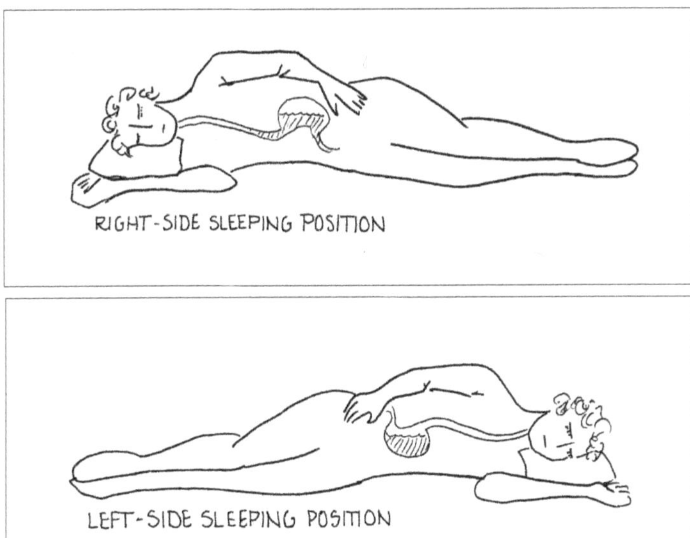

Fig. 8.1. Relationship between sleep position and reflux.

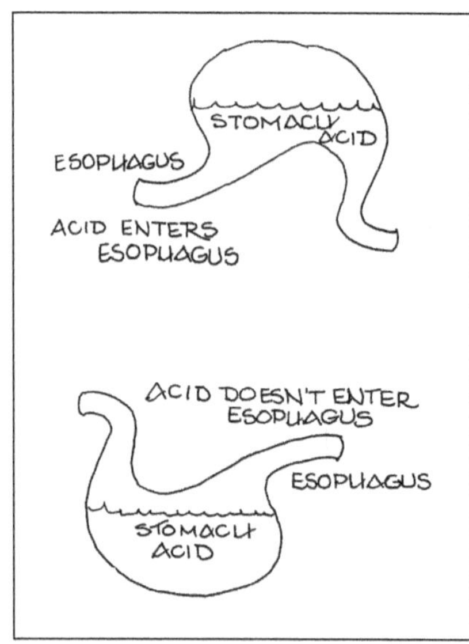

Fig. 8.2. Top: sleeping on the right side, acid enters esophagus. Bottom: Sleeping on the left side, acid does not enter esophagus.

In a recent study of 57 subjects, pH impedance testing was used to evaluate clearance of acid from the esophagus in various spontaneous sleep positions. Clearance was twice as fast sleeping on the left side compared to sleeping **supine**. Sleeping on the right side slowed the clearance even more than supine (Schuitenmaker JM, 2021). There is a reflux smartwatch app that can be used to train yourself to sleep on the left side.

From homeopathic research we know that some people find it nearly impossible to sleep on the left side. For some, sleeping on the left side may cause rapid heartrate or palpitations. In such cases, if sleeping supine is possible, it would be better than sleeping on the right with respect to reflux. Elevating the head of the bed by six inches significantly reduces esophageal acid levels in subjects with laryngopharyngeal reflux (Scott DR, 2015).

A 2021 **systematic review** evaluated five research studies that used either sleeping on a wedge pillow or elevating the head end of the bed with blocks. "The four studies that reported on GERD symptoms found an improvement among participants in the head-of-bed elevation; a high-quality **crossover trial** showed a clinically important reduction in symptom scores at six weeks and less acidic esophageal pH readings. Although the researchers suspected some of the findings less reliable, they determined elevating the head of the bed to be a cheaper and safer alternative to drug interventions (Albarqouni L, 2021)

Compared to lying on the right side, these sleep positions significantly reduce reflux:
- *Left side*
- *Supine*
- *Wedge pillow*
- *Elevating the head end of the bed by six inches*

CITATIONS

Wang SE et al, Diet and risk of gastro-oesophageal reflux disease in the Melbourne Collaborative Cohort Study, Public Health Nutr. 2021 Oct;24(15):5034-5046. PMID: 33472714

Agrawal A, Tutuian R, Hila A, Freeman J, Castell DO. Ingestion of acidic foods mimics gastroesophageal reflux during pH monitoring. Dig Dis Sci 2005; 50: 1916–20.   PMID: 16187197

Shoenut JP, Duerksen D, Yaffe CS. Impact of ingested liquids on 24-hour ambulatory pH tests. Dig Dis Sci 1998; 43: 834–9. PMID: 9558041

Pouderoux P, Friedman N, Shirazi P, Ringelstein JG, Keshavarzian A. Effect of carbonated water on gastric emptying and intragastric meal distribution. Dig Dis Sci 1997; 42: 34–9. PMID: 9009113

Kim J et al, Association between coffee intake and gastroesophageal reflux disease: a meta-analysis. Diseases of the Esophagus (2014) 27, 311–317. PMID: 23795898

Papakonstantinou E et al, Acute effects of coffee consumption on self-reported gastrointestinal symptoms, blood pressure and stress indices in healthy individuals. Nutr J. 2016; 15: 26. PMID: 26979712

Surdea-Blaga et al, Food and Gastroesophageal Reflux Disease. Curr Med Chem. 2019;26(19):3497-3511. PMID: 28521699

Kaltenbach T, Crockett S, Gerson LB, Are lifestyle measures effective in patients with gastroesophageal reflux disease? An evidence-based approach. Arch Intern Med. 2006 May 8;166(9):965-71. PMID: 16682569

Andrici J, Cox, MR, Eslick GD, Cigarette smoking and the risk of Barrett's esophagus: a systematic review and meta-analysis. J Gastroenterol Hepatol 2013 Aug;28(8):1258-73. PMID: 23611750

Dinc ASK, Cayonu M, Sengezer T, Sahim, MM, Smoking Cessation Improves the Symptoms and the Findings of Laryngeal Irritation. Ear Nose Throat J. 2020 Feb;99(2):124-127. PMID: 31608685

Kahrilas PJ, Cigarette smoking and gastroesophageal reflux disease. Dig Dis. 1992;10(2):61-71. PMID: 1591872

Ness-Jensen E, Lagergren J, Tobacco smoking, alcohol consumption and gastro-oesophageal reflux disease. Best Pract Res Clin Gastroenterol. 2017 Oct;31(5):501-508. PMID: 29195669

Franke A, Teyssen S, Singer MV, Alcohol-related diseases of the esophagus and stomach. Dig Dis. 2005;23(3-4):204-13. PMID: 16508284

Pan J, Cen L, Chen W, Yu C et al, Alcohol Consumption and the Risk of Gastroesophageal Reflux Disease: A Systematic Review and Meta-analysis. Alcohol Alcohol. 2019 Jan 1;54(1):62-69. PMID: 30184159

Langella C et al, New food approaches to reduce and/or eliminate increased gastric acidity related to gastroesophageal pathologies. Nutrition. 2018 Oct;54:26-32. PMID: 29729504

Zografos GN et al, Drug-induced esophagitis. Dis Esophagus. 2009;22(8):633-7. PMID: 19392845

Surdea-Blaga T, Negrutiu DE, Palage M, Dumitrascu DL, Food and Gastroesophageal Reflux Disease. Curr Med Chem. 2019;26(19):3497-3511. PMID: 28521699

DiSilvestro RA, Verbruggen MA, Offutt EJ, Anti-heartburn effects of a fenugreek fiber product. Phytother Res. 2011 Jan;25(1):88-91. PMID: 20623611

Morozov S, Isakov V, Konovalova M, Fiber-enriched diet helps to control symptoms and improves esophageal motility in patients with non-erosive gastroesophageal reflux disease. World J Gastroenterol. 2018 Jun 7; 24(21): 2291–2299. PMID: 29881238

Zhou C et al, Fenugreek attenuates obesity-induced inflammation and improves insulin resistance through downregulation of iRhom2/TACE. Life Sci. 2020 Oct 1;258:118222. PMID: 32768577

Pointer SD et al, Dietary Carbohydrate Intake, Insulin Resistance, and Gastroesophageal Reflux Disease (GERD): A Pilot Study in European- and African-American Obese Women. Aliment Pharmacol Ther. 2016 Nov;44(9):976-988. PMID: 27582035

Wildi AM, Tutuian R, O Castell D, The influence of rapid food intake on postprandial reflux: studies in healthy volunteers. Am J Gastroenterol. 2004 Sep;99(9):1645-51. PMID: 15330896

Kahrilas PJ, Shi G, Manka M, Joehl RJ, Increased frequency of transient lower esophageal sphincter relaxation induced by gastric distention in reflux patients with hiatal hernia. Gastroenterology. 2000 Apr;118(4):688-95. PMID: 10734020

Hsu C-S et al, Increasing insulin resistance is associated with increased severity and prevalence of gastro-oesophageal reflux disease. Aliment Pharmacol Ther. 2011 Oct;34(8):994-1004. PMID: 21848629

Corley DA, Kubo A, Body mass index and gastroesophageal reflux disease: a systematic review and meta-analysis. Am J Gastroenterol. 2006 Nov;101(11):2619-28. PMID: 16952280

Hampel H, Abraham NS, El-Serag HB, Meta-analysis: obesity and the risk for gastroesophageal reflux disease and its complications. Ann Intern Med. 2005 Aug 2;143(3):199-211. PMID: 16061918

Singh S et al, Central adiposity is associated with increased risk of esophageal inflammation, metaplasia, and adeno-carcinoma: a systematic review and meta-analysis. Clin Gastroenterol Hepatol. 2013 Nov;11(11):1399-1412.e7. PMID 23707461

Rubenstein JH et al, Protective role of gluteofemoral obesity in erosive oesophagitis and Barrett's oesophagus. Gut. 2014 Feb;63(2):230-5. PMID 23461896

Kendall BJ et al, Inverse Association Between Gluteofemoral Obesity and Risk of Barrett's Esophagus in a Pooled Analysis, Clin Gastroenterol Hepatol. 2016 Oct;14(10):1412-1419.e3. PMID 27264393

Zhang M, Hou Z-K, Huang Z-B, Chen X-L et al. Dietary and Lifestyle Factors Related to Gastroesophageal Reflux Disease: A Systematic Review. Ther Clin Risk Mana. 2021 Apr 15;17:305-323. PMID: 23707461

Randhawa MA et al, An old dietary regimen as a new lifestyle change for Gastro esophageal reflux disease: A pilot study. Pak J Pharm Sci. 2015 Sep;28(5):1583-6. PMID: 26408867

Schuitenmaker JM et al, Associations Between Sleep Position and Nocturnal Gastroesophageal Reflux: A Study Using Concurrent Monitoring of Sleep Position and Esophageal pH and Impedance. Am J Gastroenterol. 2021 Dec 20. PMID: 34928874

Scott DR, Simon RA, Supraesophageal Reflux: Correlation of Position and Occurrence of Acid Reflux-Effect of Head-of-Bed Elevation on Supine Reflux, J Allergy Clin Immunol Pract. May-Jun 2015;3(3):356-61. PMID: 25609349

Albarqouni L et al, Head of bed elevation to relieve gastroesophageal reflux symptoms: a systematic review. BMC Fam Pract. 2021; 22: 24. PMID: 33468060

Eherer A et al. Management of Gastroesophageal Reflux Disease: Lifestyle Modification and Alternative Approaches. Dig Dis 2014;32:1490151. PMID: 24603400

Homko CJ et al, Effect of dietary fat and food consistency on gastroparesis symptoms in patients with gastroparesis. Neurogastroenterol Motil. 2015 Apr;27(4):501-8. PMID: 25600163

Ebrahimpour-Koujan S, Keshteli AH, Esmaillzadeh A, Adibi P, Association between Dietary Fat Intake and Odds of Gastro-esophageal Reflux Disorder (GERD) in Iranian Adults. Int J Prev Med. 2021 Jul 5;12:77. PMID: 34447519

Rajaie S et al, Spicy Food Consumption and Risk of Uninvestigated Heartburn in Isfahani Adults. Dig Dis. 2020;38(3):178-187. PMID: 31473738

Gonlachanvit S, Are rice and spicy diet good for functional gastrointestinal disorders? J Neurogastroenterol Motil. 2010 Apr;16(2):131-8. PMID: 20535343

Vora A, Vance D, Alnouri G, Sataloff RT, Food Sensitivity and Laryngopharyngeal Reflux: Preliminary Observations. J Voice. 2021 May;35(3):497.e5-497. PMID: 31685326

NINE

DIETS FOR THE TREATMENT OF REFLUX

Your diet affects how your body works
And can cause or allay mucosal fits and jerks.
To be reprieved
From what has aggrieved,
Eat what's right for your body's quirks.

GLOSSARY

demulcent—a substance that relieves irritation of mucous membranes by forming a protective film

glycosaminoglycans—complex sugars occurring chiefly as components of connective tissue such as cartillage

migrating motor complex—a cyclic, recurring muscle contraction pattern occurring in the stomach and small bowel during fasting; it is interrupted by eating.

KEY QUESTIONS

What are the details of various dietary approaches to reducing reflux?

Can dietary changes cure reflux?

While this chapter will describe the variety of dietary programs I have successfully used in the treatment of GERD, I feel the best approach is to work with a qualified and experienced nutritionist who can tailor some aspects of these diets to the individual.

I have found that diet and nutrition are key features in resolving or reducing symptoms of reflux. The amount and type of carbohydrate in the diet can be a major factor (Pointer SD, 2016). In a four-month study of 42 obese women with GERD, a high fat, low carbohydrate diet significantly reduced symptoms and use of medication. A smaller study also found improved symptoms as well as reduction of the esophageal acid exposure time after just one week on a low carbohydrate diet (Austin GL, 2006).

Until the late 1980s, certain classic conditions now known to be associated with diet were virtually ignored by most of conventional medicine. For instance, celiac disease was rarely considered worthy of being part of the diagnostic workup for GI symptoms. Celiac was considered a rare condition with an estimated prevalence of 0.03% of the U.S. population (Lohi S, 2007). Because of this skewed belief, the diagnosis typically was made only after an average of ten years of medical visits. Now we know that celiac disease affects at least 1% of the population. Diagnostic testing for celiac disease is now part of a standard GI workup (Dubé C, 2005).

Much has changed with respect to diet in mainstream medicine. The FODMAP diet is well researched for IBS and most physicians recognize its value. The Specific Carbohydrate Diet has also been the subject of initial studies published in respected peer reviewed journals.

For more information and links to the diets discussed below, see Dr. Allison Siebecker's excellent website at https://www.siboinfo.com/diet.html

The Specific Carbohydrate Diet (SCD)

The specific carbohydrate diet was developed by Sidney Haas, a pediatric gastroenterologist, in the 1930's and published in 1951 (Kakodkar S, 2015). The purpose of the diet is to reduce the amount of fermentable carbohydrate to prevent overgrowth of normal intestinal bacteria and archaea. It allows the simplest types of sugars (monosaccharides) while excluding more complex sugars (disaccharides and most polysaccharides). The complex sugars are harder for humans to digest and therefore can promote microbial growth. SCD is not appropriate for vegans or more limited vegetarian diets. Yogurt fermented for 24 hours is lactose-free and an important component of the diet when tolerated. Commercial yogurt is fermented for six to eight hours which allows exposure to traces of lactose (a disaccharide sugar not permitted on SCD). Full 24-hour fermentation converts all the lactose to lactic acid. This diet does not include starchy vegetables and grains. For those who are underweight, I often modify it by adding white rice, winter squash, increased fat, and other specific foods to prevent weight loss.

To prevent overgrowth of gut microorganisms, the Specific Carbohydrate Diet reduces the amount of fermentable carbohydrate.

24-hour yogurt is allowed because it is lactose-free.

The SCD is designed to promote restoration of a healthy microbiome and has been studied as an important part of the treatment in inflammatory bowel diseases (IBD).

TABLE 9.1. SPECIFIC CARBOHYDRATE DIET FOODS (SCD)	
Compliant Foods	**Noncompliant Foods**
Vegetables—except for okra, white potato, yam, sweet potato, and parsnip	Sucrose
Fruits	Maltose
Nut flours	Isomaltose
Certain soaked and home-cooked beans—navy, lima and lentils (Burgis JC, 2016)	Lactose
Dry curd cottage cheese	Grains
Firm cheeses (aged at least 30 days)	Potatoes
Meat	Okra
Poultry	Parsnip
Fish	Corn
Eggs	Fluid milk
Honey (Obih C, 2016)	Soy
Butter	High lactose cheeses, such as soft cheese, fermented less than 30 days
Oils	Processed meats
	Canned food and dietary additives/preservatives

Low **FODMAP** Diet

FODMAP foods are rapidly fermented by bacteria, leading to symptoms of gas, distention, altered motility and abdominal pain. In part because of increased fructose consumption in the form of fruit juice and high fructose corn syrup, intake of FODMAP foods has increased in Western diets.

The term FODMAP was originally coined by Monash University in Melbourne, Australia (Dugum M, 2016). The mnemonic stands for:

> F – fermentable
>
> O – oligosaccharides
>
> D – disaccharides
>
> M – monosaccharides
>
> A - and
>
> P- polyols

Fermentable Carbohydrates

FODMAP foods are poorly absorbed fermentable carbohydrates (prebiotics) that, in excess, can cause increased TSLERs which were discussed in chapter three (Piche T, 2003 and Geysen H, 2020). Recall that TSLERs contribute to GERD because the LES is relaxed for longer periods. High FODMAP foods can also cause intestinal problems by drawing water into the small and large intestines. These prebiotics may also feed the microbes in the small intestine, increasing gas production. More gas increases pressure and symptoms in small intestine bacterial overgrowth (SIBO). The Low FODMAP diet has been shown to be effective in as many as 74% of patients with IBS, reducing the symptoms of bloating, nausea, abdominal pain, and diarrhea (Nanayakkara WS, 2016, Marsh A, 2016, Rao SS, 2015, Chumpitazi BP, 2015). This diet has also been used to reduce symptoms in inflammatory bowel diseases (Popa SL, 2020, Cox SR, 2020).

OLIGOSACCHARIDES

Oligosaccharides include fructo-oligosaccharides, fructans (such as inulin) and galacto-oligosaccharides.

Galacto-oligosaccharides are fermented in the colon because humans do not have an enzyme to digest and absorb them higher in the GI tract.

Examples include:

- Legumes
- Some nuts and seeds
- Some grains
- Dairy products
- Human milk
- Some commercial infant formulas

DISACCHARIDES

Disaccharides include lactose, sucrose, maltose, and trehalose. Lactose is poorly absorbed in lactase deficiency and, as discussed under SCD, feeds small intestine microbes in patients with SIBO. Up to 70% of the world's inhabitants have primary lactose deficiency (aka lactose intolerance). Typical onset is between ages two and six.

Sources include:

- Dairy products that are not fully fermented
- Possible additives in breads, cakes, diet products

MONOSACCHARIDES

The major source of monosaccharide is fructose. It is absorbed easily in the small bowel. One of the mechanisms for absorption requires the presence of glucose for activation. If more fructose than glucose is present, some fructose may not be absorbed, feeding the small bowel bacteria. Some people have actual fructose malabsorption, but the accuracy of fructose breath tests to diagnose this condition have been debated (Putkonen L, 2016),

Fructose sources include:

- Fruit

- Fruit products

- Honey

- High-fructose corn syrup, a major component of many processed foods

In practice, I have found that fructose intolerance is less common than lactose intolerance.

I suggest starting the full Low FODMAP diet initially, but because I find that true fructose intolerance is not as common as lactose intolerance, I have found that gradual reintroduction of lower and moderate FODMAP fruits and honey may prove to be well tolerated.

According to the Monash University website (www. monashfodmap.com), low FODMAP sweeteners include sucrose, maple syrup and rice malt syrup.

Sucrose (table sugar) is a disaccharide digested by the enzyme sucrase, releasing fructose and glucose. Honey is a liquid solution of fructose and glucose which requires no enzyme for digestion. Many patients tolerate honey unless they have a distinct fructose malabsorption syndrome.

POLYOLS

Polyols are sugar-alcohols which include mannitol, xylitol, erythritol and sorbitol.

Polyol sources include:

- Certain fruits (e.g., plums) & vegetables (e.g., cauliflower, mushrooms)

- Sugar-free chewing gum & other "sugar-free" or "diet" foods

IMPLEMENTATION AND DRAWBACKS

A Monash University smart phone application is a useful source of up-to-date information on the FODMAP content of various foods. FODMAP intake has an additive effect, which means the more one eats, the greater the symptoms. Considering the total FODMAP intake per meal is important for symptom reduction.

The diet is implemented in two phases: An elimination phase for six to eight weeks is followed by gradual reintroduction once symptoms are controlled. Transition to a less restrictive version of the diet is the goal because prebiotics are necessary for the health of the beneficial colonic microbiota. Slowly reintroducing moderate portions of these foods while monitoring for an increase in symptoms is key to individualizing the diet during this latter phase. Because of the inclusion of grains, I find that this diet, or the Cedars-Sinai diet, is the best choice for strict vegetarians or vegans. Websites for vegan friendly FODMAP diet guidelines may be useful for these patients.

Possible drawbacks of the Low FODMAP diet include difficulties with adherence, risk of reduction in colonic bacteria, reduced total fiber intake and deficient calcium intake. If tolerated, the addition of lactose-free dairy products (discussed above in the SCD section) provides a good source of calcium and protein.

SIBO Specific Food Guide (SSFG)

I rely on this diet plan to:

1. reduce symptoms in reflux

2. induce remission in IBD (Crohn's, ulcerative colitis, and microscopic colitis)

3. treat celiac disease or non-celiac gluten intolerance that is non-responsive to a standard gluten-free diet

4. prevent recurrence of SIBO after effective treatment

I tell my student physicians that giving a patient two different diets to follow is not a good idea because it leads to confusion and excessive restriction of food choices.

Allison Siebecker, ND, has done a great service by creating a synthesis of the low FODMAP diet, the SCD, some aspects of the Cedars-Sinai diet and her own clinical experience with SIBO/IBS patients. It is an excellent first choice for treatment of IBD, IBS, celiac disease and SIBO or for those who have not had sufficient symptomatic relief from trials of other diets. A colorful chart of this guide is available at no charge at www.siboinfo.com under the treatment/diet dropdown menu. The SSFG encourages the use of carbohydrates that are easily absorbed in the upper small intestine. Because they are readily absorbed, they are less likely to increase gas production and pressure that can cause reflux. It is lower in starch, fiber, and fermentable fruits and vegetables.

The SSFG encourages the use of carbohydrates that are easily absorbed in the upper small intestine.

SSFG Guidelines

Although garlic and onion are high FODMAP and there-fore not part of this diet, the upper portion of the green onion is often well tolerated.

Strained garlic infused oil may be used in cooking because the problematic fructans in garlic remain in the solids of the garlic clove.

- Begin with no beans or raw foods for sensitive patients (these can be added later)

- Begin with peeled, de-seeded vegetables and fruits for sensitive patients

- Allow at least 4 hours between meals and a 12 hour fast overnight to allow the migrating motor complex (MMC) to function optimally, although this may not be appropriate for those who are underweight or have unstable blood sugar levels.

Foods avoided

- Grains
- Sweeteners other than honey or liquid stevia extract
- Corn, soy, tubers
- Thickeners—carrageenan, guar gum, xanthan gum
- Mucilaginous foods—flax, chia, seaweed, okra, and demul-cent herbs
- Beans (lentils, navy and lima beans may be added progres-sively)

Foods permitted with unlimited use (Ong DK, 2010)

- Fowl, fish, eggs, and red meat
- Fat
- Lactose-free dairy (if casein is tolerated)
    - Ghee
    - Aged cheeses
    - 24-hour yogurt

    To provide a higher calorie content for underweight patients, a base of 50:50 milk/cream may be used.

    For casein sensitivity, a base of coconut milk without added gum thickeners may be use in place of mamma-lian milk.

- Low FODMAP Vegetables

    Unlimited per FODMAP quantity restrictions or Dr. Siebeck-er's clinical experience.

Although garlic and onion are high FODMAP and therefore not part of this diet, the upper portion of the green onion is often well tolerated. Strained garlic infused oil may be used in cooking because the problematic fructans in garlic remain in the solids of the garlic clove. Garlic powder cannot be used on this diet.

- Low FODMAP fruits
- Most nuts and seeds
- Winter squash

Foods with special explanations

- Honey, liquid stevia, and some fruit juices as sweetemers

    Typically excluded on the FODMAP diet, but permitted on SIBO Specific Food Guide

    Certain varieties (for example, clover honey) have been permitted on the premise that they have a favorable glucose to fructose ratio and therefore are low FODMAP

- Bone broth

    Bone broth made from whole bones is not permitted due to the glycosaminoglycans sugar compounds found in cartilage.

    Bone broth made from marrow bones (bone shaft without the joint cartilage) is permitted

Consider individualizing the diet. While most patients can tolerate the following five categories, they may cause problems for some people. I call these the "high five" *

- Dairy
- Eggs
- Raw fruits and vegetables
- Too much fruit or honey
- Nuts and seeds

After several months of remission, one may carefully reintroduce, one at a time, moderate and eventually high FODMAPs items—with a careful eye for aggravation of symptoms. Working with a knowledgeable SSFG physician or nutritionist is strongly advised for best results during all phases of the diet.

CEDARS-SINAI/LOW FERMENTATION DIET

Dr. Mark Pimentel and his team at Cedars-Sinai medical center developed a dietary protocol for prevention of relapse after successful treatment of SIBO. It may relieve reflux as well (Pimentel M, 2006). Of all the diets described in this chapter,

---

*This is a slight expansion of a concept from scdlifestyle.com originally and colorfully called "the four horsemen of the apocalypse".

this is the simplest to follow and supports the broadest choice of foods. It is a good choice for vegetarians, vegans and patients who do not want many dietary restrictions. It is a useful guide when traveling because it has a broader choice of foods than the other diets. Those with a history of disordered eating may find the Cedars-Sinai diet preferable to more restrictive diets. If you have a history of disordered eating, please discuss any dietary changes with your counselor and nutritionist before starting a new program.

Key features are:

- Food timing to promote motility

  The recommendation is to space meals at least 4-5 hours apart to allow migrating motor complex production of "cleansing waves/housekeeping waves" in the small intestine. Therefore, snacking between meals and at bedtime is discouraged.

- Low carbohydrate

  This approach limits the quantity of starches but allows most grains, potato, etc.

  Permitted sugars = sucrose, glucose, aspartame (Nutra Sweet)

  Total sugar intake is limited to less than 40 grams per day

  Most hard-to-digest sugars are eliminated: fructose (such as high fructose corn syrup), lactose, sucralose (Splenda), sugar alcohols such as sorbitol, xylitol, mannitol, erythritol, lactulose, and lactitol (https://www.gidoctor.net/contents/diet-for-ibs-and-sibo)

Other permitted foods

- Lactase treated milk products and non-dairy milk (check if the latter is sweetened)

    Lactaid milk

    Almond milk

    Rice milk

- Carbohydrates—limit to ½ -1 cup serving per meal

    White rice

    Potatoes

    Sweet Potatoes

    White bread (sourdough, Italian, French, potato)

    Rice Krispies cereal

    White pasta

    Cream of wheat hot breakfast cereal

- Nuts
- Chocolate (as stated in chapter 6, for some this may trigger heartburn)
- Meat/seafood/eggs - chicken, pork, beef, fish, eggs
- Whey protein powder (and other protein powders not sweetened with prohibited sugars)
- Fats
- Most vegetables

    Moderate use of raw vegetables/small salads

    Peppers, tomatoes, cucumber, zucchini, squash, eggplant, peas (but not the edible pod). These vegetables are considered more "fruit-like vegetables" due to their botanical type (prominent seeds; grown above ground)

    Vegetables that grow underground: onions, garlic, beets, carrots, turnips, etc. (for some, spices such as garlic and onions may trigger reflux)

    Recommended daily intake of cooked vegetables—3-5 cups

- Most fruits—limited to 2 servings/day

    Fresh fruits rather than dried fruit

- Coffee

    1-2 cups daily (as with chocolate, coffee may trigger heartburn for some)

Foods excluded

- Probiotic-rich foods (such as yogurt)
- Dairy products—cheese, non-lactase treated milk, butter, yogurt
- Chewing gum or other products containing sugar alcohols
- High fiber foods and supplements

> Metamucil
>
> Oatmeal
>
> Wild rice
>
> Whole wheat or multigrain breads

- Beans/legumes—hummus, lentils, peas, soy products (tofu, soymilk) etc.
- Cabbage, brussels sprouts, broccoli, cauliflower, larger portions of leafy vegetables
- Eat, but limit: apples, pears, bananas
- Fruit juice

FAST TRACT DIET

(Norm Robillard, PhD) (https://digestivehealthinstitute.org)

This is an exchange system that uses a point scale to choose foods. It is a low fermentation diet as are all the diets in this chapter but is based on Dr. Robillard's experience and research into the effect of various carbohydrate foods on reflux. An app and a book entitled *Fast Tract Digestion—Heartburn* are available at his website.

CITATIONS

Pointer SD, Rickstrew J, Slaughter JC, Vaezi MF, Silver HJ. Dietary carbohydrate intake, insulin resistance and gastro-oesophageal re-flux disease: a pilot study in European- and African-American obese women. Aliment Pharmacol Ther. 2016;44(9):976–88. PMID: 27582035

Austin GL, Thiny MT, Westman EC, Yancy WS Jr, Shaheen NJ. A very low-carbohydrate diet improves gastroesophageal reflux and its symptoms. Dig Dis Sci. 2006;51(8):1307–12. PMID: 16871438

Lohi S, Mustalahti K, Kaukinen K, Laurila K et al. Increasing prevalence of coeliac disease over time. Aliment Pharmacol Ther. 2007 Nov 1;26(9):1217-25. PMID: 17944736

Dube C, Rostom A, Sy R, Cranney A et al. The prevalence of celiac disease in average-risk and at-risk Western European populations: a systematic review. Gastroenterology. 2005 Apr;128(4 Suppl 1):S57-67. PMID: 15825128

Kakodkar S, Farooqui AJ, Mikolaitis SL, Mutlu EA. The Specific Carbohydrate Diet for Inflammatory Bowel Disease: A Case Series. J Acad Nutr Diet. 2015;115(8):1226-32. PMID: 26210084

Burgis JC, Nguyen K, Park KT, Cox K. Response to strict and liberalized specific carbohydrate diet in pediatric Crohn's disease. World J Gastroenterol. 2016;22(6):2111-7. PMID: 26877615

Obih C, Wahbeh G, Lee D, et al. Specific carbohydrate diet for pediatric inflammatory bowel disease in clinical practice within an academic IBD center. Nutrition. 2016;32(4):418-25. PMID: 26655069

Dugum M, Barco K, Garg S. Managing irritable bowel syndrome: The low-FODMAP diet. Cleve Clin J Med. 2016;83(9):655-62. PMID: 27618353

Piche T et al, Colonic fermentation influences lower esophageal sphincter function in gastroesophageal reflux disease. Gastroenterology.2003 Apr;124(4):894-902. PMID: 12671885

Geyson H et al, Acute administration of fructans increases the number of transient lower esophageal sphincter relaxations in healthy volunteers. Neurogastroenterol Motil . 2020 Jan;32(1):e13727. PMID: 12671885

Khandalavala BN, Nirmalraj MC. Resolution of Severe Ulcerative Colitis with the Specific Carbohydrate Diet. Case Rep Gastroenterol. 2015;9(2):291-5. PMID: 26351419

Nanayakkara WS, Skidmore PM, O'brien L, Wilkinson TJ, Gearry RB. Efficacy of the low FODMAP diet for treating irritable bowel syndrome: the evidence to date. Clin Exp Gastroenterol. 2016;9:131-42. PMID: 27382323

Marsh A, Eslick EM, Eslick G, Does a diet low in FODMAPs reduce symptoms associated with functional gastrointestinal disorders? A comprehensive systematic review and meta-analysis. Eur J Nutr. 2016 Apr;55(3):897-906. PMID: 25982757

Rao SS, Yu S, Fedewa A. A Systematic review: dietary fibre and FODMAP-restricted diet in the management of constipation and irritable bowel syndrome

Aliment Pharmacol Ther. 2015 Jun;41(12):1256-70. PMID: 25903636

Chumpitazi BP, Cope JL, Hollister EB, et al. Randomised clinical trial: gut microbiome biomarkers are associated with clinical response to a low FODMAP diet in children with the irritable bowel syndrome. Aliment Pharmacol Ther. 2015;42(4):418-27. PMID: 26104013

Putkonen L, Yao CK, Gibson PR. Fructose malabsorption syndrome, Curr Opin Clin Nutr Metab Care. 2013 Jul;16(4):473-7. PMID: 23739630

Popa SL, Pop C, Dumitrascu DL. Diet Advice for Crohn's Disease: FODMAP and Beyond. Nutrients. 2020 Dec 6;12(12):3751. PMID: 33291329

Cox SR, Lindsay JO, Fromentin S, Stagg AJ, et al. Effects of Low FODMAP Diet on Symptoms, Fecal Microbiome, and Markers of Inflammation in Patients With Quiescent Inflammatory Bowel Disease in a Randomized Trial. Gastroenterology. 2020 Jan;158(1):176-188.e7. PMID: 31586453

Ong DK, Mitchell SB, Barrett JS, et al. Manipulation of dietary short chain carbohydrates alters the pattern of gas production and genesis of symptoms in irritable bowel syndrome. J Gastroenterol Hepatol. 2010;25(8):1366-73. PMID: 20659225

https://www.gidoctor.net/contents/diet-for-ibs-and-sibo

Pimentel M, Pimentel MA. A New IBS Solution, Bacteria-the Missing Link in Treating Irritable Bowel Syndrome. Sherman Oaks, CA : Health Point Press, 2006.

TEN

NATURAL REMEDIES FOR REFLUX

To strengthen mucosal defense,
Zinc, ginger, and demulcents.
Quercetin, limonene,
And turmeric will be seen,
To offer protection immense.

GLOSSARY

antispasmodic—medicinal substances that relieve muscle cramping

carminative—herbal medicines that reduce gas production or help expel it

cephalic (head) phase of digestion—the phase of digestion that starts with the brain even before the food is eaten

demulcents—medicinal substances that coat and soothe

hypochlorhydria—decreased levels of acid in the stomach

prokinetic—a medicinal substance that increases the downward movement through the GI tract

strictures—bands of fibrous tissue within hollow organs such as the digestive tract

KEY QUESTIONS

What are the research-proven natural medicines for GERD?

Which causes of reflux do the various treatments address?

Patients are encouraged to discuss these natural remedies with knowledgeable healthcare professionals to determine individual appropriateness, dosages, and drug-nutrient-herbal interactions.

In 2018 an online survey conducted by the Division of Gastroenterology at the University of Pennsylvania found that the rate of alternative medicine use among patients with gastrointestinal disorders was as high as 85% (Yoon SL, 2018). It is clear people are looking for help beyond what they are receiving in standard practice medicine. There is a wide range of nutritional, herbal, and prescription medicines that I use to treat my patients. These options allow the various causes of reflux to be addressed. Several natural remedies benefit people with GERD through multiple mechanisms. For example, melatonin is thought to improve sphincter tone, protect against **free radical damage**, and modify gastric acid production.

I have organized this chapter by treatments for various underlying causes, so you will notice herbal, nutritional and drug therapies combined rather than isolated into separate sections. It is organized much like chapter three.

TREATMENTS TO ENHANCE ESOPHAGEAL DEFENSE FACTORS

Licorice Root

Demulcents are plants that form a soothing film. Deglycyrrhizinated licorice (DGL) is a licorice extract without any of the blood pressure or water retention effects that higher doses of whole licorice root have. DGL is available in capsules, chewable tablets, and as a powder. DGL may be combined with other ingredients which may be problematic if they contain polyols or fructose. There is little published research on DGL and esophagitis. Aspirin and bile are extremely irritating to the esophagus and stomach. A study found that when DGL was given by mouth to rats along with aspirin or bile, it reduced the anticipated damage to the esophagus (Russell RI, 1984). DGL increased the number of mucus producing cells in the upper stomach as well as total mucus production (van Marle J, 1981).

Other demulcent herbs include slippery elm (*Ulmus rubra*), marshmallow root (*Althea officinalis*), and aloe (*Aloe vera*).

Aloe Vera

Aloe vera juice was found to be as effective in reducing symptoms as omeprazole (PPI) or ranitidine (an H2 antagonist) in a 4-week randomized controlled trial of 79 subjects with GERD (Panahi Y, 2015).

Zinc Carnosine

This form of zinc is described as an antioxidant, anti-inflammatory, and vulnerary (promotes wound healing). It reduced **stricture** formation and tissue damage in bleach-induced esophageal burns (Ozbayoglu A, 2017) as well as alcohol induced damage to the stomach lining. As an oral rinse, it was found to prevent mouth sores in patients undergoing head and neck radiation for oral cancer treatment (Hewlings S, 2020). It reduced the risk of developing painful ulcers and aided healing of ulcers that did form in patients receiving chemotherapy and radiation therapy (Hayashi H, 2014). Zinc carnosine mixed with sodium alginate, a seaweed extract, was given to lung cancer patients during chemo-radiation therapy to prevent esophagitis (Yanase K, 2015). Compared to receiving sodium alginate alone, the addition of zinc carnosine reduced the incidence of esophagitis by almost 40%.

Quercetin

A study compared the protective effects of quercetin and vitamin E against reflux esophagitis to that of omeprazole (a PPI). Rats received either a single dose of quercetin and α-tocopherol (vitamin E), or one dose of omeprazole one hour prior to surgery. Quercetin and α-tocopherol significantly prevented rats from developing esophagitis compared to the PPI. The quercetin and vitamin E treated rats also had higher protective antioxidant levels in their tissues (**catalase, superoxide dismutase** and **glutathione**). Quercetin also significantly lowered blood levels of proinflammatory histamine (Rao CV, 2008).

Curcumin

Curcumin is an extract of turmeric. Research shows that turmeric reduces inflammation, decreases free radical tissue damage, prevents death of healthy cells, reduces risk of developing cancer, and may prevent certain cancers from metastatic spread through the body (Kwiecien S, 2019). In rats, turmeric extract was effective, but not as effective as lansoprazole (a proton pump inhibitor) in preventing acute reflux esophagitis. It was more effective than lansoprazole in preventing mixed bile and acid reflux esophagitis (Mahattanadul S, 2006).

In another study, 16 Barrett's esophagus patients took 500 mg of curcumin daily the week prior to an upper endoscopy exam. Compared to 17 Barrett's patients who did not take the curcumin, biopsies showed moderately reduced inflammatory activity. Even more impressive was a doubling of **apoptosis** of abnormal Barrett's cells (Rawat N, 2012).

Melatonin

Melatonin controls blood flow in the vessels of the mucus membranes of the upper digestive tract (Konturek SJ, 2007 and Majka J, 2018). It protects the esophagus and stomach from the damaging effects of acid, pepsin, and bile (Madalinski MH, 2011). For more details, see chapter six.

D-limonene

D-limonene is an oil found in orange, lemon, mandarin, lime, kumquat, and grapefruit. It is used as a flavoring in common processed foods. As a natural medicine it is used to treat reflux by stimulating protective mucus, reducing inflammatory chemicals (**PGE2** and **nitrates**) and healing erosions and ulcers (Moraes TM, 2013). It has been used as a **prokinetic**, improving motility and peristalsis in the upper digestive tract. It also is used to treat cholesterol containing gallstones and has been proven to increase levels of certain enzymes that detoxify carcinogens (Anandakumar P, 2020).

TREATMENTS TO IMPROVE LAX **LES** / REDUCED **LES** PRESSURE AND TRANSIENT LOWER ESOPHAGEAL SPHINCTER RELAXATIONS (TLESRs)

As discussed in chapter three, the LES is triggered to open momentarily when the wave of muscular peristalsis brings a bolus of swallowed food to the stomach. The LES requires good muscle tone at all stages of its activity except for the short period of relaxation needed to allow the bolus to pass into the stomach. TLESRs are periods of LES relaxation that allow for gas to be vented from the stomach. If these relaxations are too frequent or prolonged, they increase the risk of significant reflux.

SUPPLEMENTS

Melatonin

An Egyptian study found that GERD patients treated with melatonin for one to two months had marked improvement in symptoms of heartburn and upper abdominal pain. There were also significant improvements in all the healthy activities of the lower esophageal sphincter. These activities included better muscle tone during contraction and relaxation phases and shorter relaxation times (Kandil TS, 2010). A Brazilian study found that one tablet a day comprised of a combination of melatonin (6 mg), tryptophan (200 mg), vitamin B12 (50 mcg), methionine (100 mg), vitamin B6 (25 mg), folic acid (10 mg) and betaine (100 mg/*not betaine hydrochloride*) resolved heartburn symptoms as well or better than omeprazole after 40 days. One of the proposed mechanisms for this reduction in reflux symptoms was improved LES muscle tone (Pereira, RdS, 2006).

Huperzine A

Acetylcholine is the major neurotransmitter needed for the proper function of the parasympathetic nervous system, referred to as the "rest and digest" portion of the autonomic nervous system. It has important functions throughout the body and is especially active in the gut regarding sphincter muscle tone.

Huperzia is an herb used in Argentinian traditional medicine as an aphrodisiac and for improving memory. Huperzine A is an extract of this herb. It contains acetylcholinesterase inhibitors which prevent excess breakdown of acetylcholine (Ortega MG, 2004). Most who know about this extract think of it as a treatment for improving memory, but years ago I learned it reduces reflux by improving LES tone. I am not aware of a study proving it, but I learned about it from Dr. Davis Lamson, a naturopathic physician and professor, several decades ago. I have helped several GERD patients who had laxity of the LES by using huperzine A. Two months of daily use allows time for best results. It can be continued as needed if it proves helpful.

Phosphatidylcholine (PC)

Dr. Lamson also taught me that phosphatidylcholine (also known as lecithin) may be used as a supplemental source of choline. Choline can be converted into the neurotransmitter acetylcholine. PC may further improve the function of the LES. I prefer the lecithin sourced from sunflower rather than soy.

DEVICES

IQoro

This device is placed in the mouth between the teeth and lips and used to exercise all the muscles involved in swallowing. It is used for about 40 seconds and repeated 3 times a day for a six-month period. Research shows it treats reflux including that caused by sliding hiatal hernia and has been found to work for people of all body weight classes (Hägg M, 2015 and Franzén T, 2019).

Stretta

This is a device used to improve the tone of the LES using low temperature radiofrequency energy. It is an endoscopic procedure specific for laxity of the LES. Studies show strengthening of the LES and a reduction in transient LES relaxations (Tam WC, 2003). This non-drug treatment may repair the deficient sphincter, reduce the need for acid blocking medications and have long term benefits. It is not widely available at the time of this writing.

TREATMENTS FOR DELAYED GASTRIC EMPTYING (GASTROPARESIS)

Ginger (*Zingiber officinalis*)

Two human studies done in China showed that eating ginger increases gastric emptying with the major effect being increased motility of the antrum (Wu K-L, 2008 and Hu M-L, 2011). An Italian randomized placebo controlled cross-over study found similar effects using a combination of ginger and artichoke extracts (Lazzini S, 2016). A study looking into the mechanism behind ginger's anti-nausea and prokinetic effects found that it relaxed spasms in the stomach and increased levels of the neurotransmitter acetylcholine (Ghayr MN, 2005). Ginger is proven to relieve nausea and vomiting from multiple causes including chemotherapy, motion sickness, pregnancy, or post-surgical (Bodagh MN, 2018).

Ginger reduces nausea by relaxing spasms in the stomach and increases levels of the neurotransmitter acetylcholine.

Ginger is proven to relieve nausea and vomiting.

Iberogast (Sometimes Referred To As STW 5 in Research)

Iberogast is a German herbal combination with significant prokinetic effects. Two studies compared Iberogast with the prescription prokinetics metoclopramide and cisapride and found similar therapeutic effects in the treatment of dyspepsia. Unlike the pharmaceuticals, Iberogast does not have dangerous side effects such as heart arrhythmias. Also, the combination of herbs in the formula are **carminative**, **antispasmodic**, and tonic to general digestive processes (Saller R, 2002). It may be wise to periodically test liver enzymes in patients with known liver disease who choose to take Iberogast (Gerhardt F, 2019).

I also use prescription prokinetics such as low doses of erythromycin and prucalopride (brand names Motegrity and Resolor). Erythromycin has its effects on the stomach and small intestine. Prucalopride additionally affects serotonin receptors in the colon and is used as a prokinetic and laxative.

Small Intestine Bacterial Overgrowth (SIBO)

Gut bacteria ferment carbohydrates to produce hydrogen gas. Excessive gas due to overgrowth of these bacteria leads to higher pressure below the diaphragm which may increase reflux. Natural treatments may include a low fermentation diet, berberine containing herbs such as *Hydrastis canadensis* (goldenseal), *Berberis aquafolium* (Oregon grape) and *Berberis vulgaris* (barberry). *Origanum vulgare* (oregano) is another effective treatment (Chedid V, 2014). The most used prescription treatment is an antibiotic called rifaximin (Xifaxan). When hydrogen levels are extremely high and other treatments have not been effective, a liquid fast called an elemental diet may be required. See chapter sixteen for more on elemental diets.

Intestinal Methanogen Overgrowth (IMO)

Methanogens are archaebacteria—organisms that covert hydrogen into methane. Either of these gases, if excessive, will increase the intra-abdominal pressure and promote reflux. Methane may be even more of a problem than hydrogen alone. Methane slows transit through the small intestine by up to 59% (Pimental M, 2006). Natural treatments to reduce the level of methanogens include a low fermentation diet, allicin (a low FODMAP extract of garlic), *Origanum vulgare* (oregano), and *Lactobacillus reuteri* DSM 17938 in the product named Biogaia Protectis Drops (Ojetti V, 2017). A combination of quebracho, peppermint, and horse chestnut (Atrantil) has been found to reduce symptoms caused by excessive methane and a current research trial is testing its effectiveness for lowering methane gas levels (Brown K, 2016, NCT04755673). A prescription treatment would include a combination of rifaximin (Xifaxan) and either metronidazole (Flagyl) or neomycin.

Hiatal Hernia

When a portion of the upper stomach moves through the hiatus of the diaphragm into the chest, it is referred to as a sliding hiatal hernia. The hernia is a small portion of the stomach extending into the chest, creating a pouch which easily refluxes stomach contents into the esophagus. In this situation, the LES and diaphragm are separated by several centimeters and can no longer work together. Treatments involve visceral massage techniques to correct small hernias, special exercises to strengthen core abdominal muscles, breathing techniques, and therapies for microbial overgrowth to reduce intra-abdominal pressure. See chapter twelve for details.

Altered pH

Hypochlorhydria is the most common finding seen during Heidelberg testing (see chapter four). The test is performed to directly measure the pH of the stomach. When hypochlorhydria is found, bitters, vinegar or betaine hydrochloride capsules can be taken during the test to measure their ability to normalize the acid levels.

Bitter Herbs

Bitter herb examples include *Gentian lutea* (gentian), *Taraxacum officinale* (dandelion), *Rumex crispus* (yellow dock) and *Citrus aurantium* (bitter orange peel). These are best taken prior to meals.

Smelling the food being prepared and thinking about the food can also increase production of acid. This is also called the **cephalic phase** of digestion.

Taking 1-2 teaspoons of apple cider vinegar mixed in two ounces of water before meals may have a beneficial effect on pH. If vinegar is used regularly, it is best to rinse the teeth with water or brush immediately after drinking the solution. Drinking the vinegar mixture through a straw will also prevent damage to dental enamel. Be aware that using fermented foods such as apple cider vinegar may aggravate heartburn or other symptoms in those with histamine intolerance. Fermentation increases the production of histamine in food and drink.

Taking apple cider vinegar in water before meals may help reduce heartburn.

Drinking the vinegar mixture through a straw helps to prevent damage to dental enamel.

Betaine hydrochloride capsules taken with meals may also provide needed acid for those with hypochlorhydria. Most formulations also contain the enzyme pepsin which works with hydrochloric acid during protein digestion in the stomach.

Hyperchlorhydria or true excess acid production is a less common finding during Heidelberg testing. It can be treated by enhancing esophageal defence factors as discussed above. In addition, melatonin may balance the production of acid. Some cases will also require treatments for histamine intolerance which may include H2 receptor antagonists such as famotidine (Pepcid AC). Others may respond to sodium alginate (products such as Heartburn Soothe) which forms a "raft" of gel on the upper surface of stomach contents thereby preventing reflux. Sodium alginate may also be effective for non-acid and weakly acid reflux. Drinking water that is treated to increase alkalinity may also be helpful (see below).

Acid Pocket

Research supports the concept of an acid pocket. This refers to a thin, highly concentrated layer of acid floating at the top of stomach contents after meals. Being at the top puts this acidic fluid closer to the esophagus which makes reflux more likely.

The most specific treatment to prevent reflux of the acid pocket is a combination of sodium alginate and an antacid. Sodium alginate is derived from seaweed. When swallowed, the powder, chewable, or liquid alginate forms a gel that floats on top of the gastric contents. This gel is described as a "raft" which is a barrier to prevent reflux. In addition, the antacid (usually calcium carbonate or sodium bicarbonate) neutralizes any acid adjacent to the gel layer. A 2019 double-blind placebo-controlled trial found this treatment significantly improved symptoms of heartburn, regurgitation, and dyspepsia (Wilkinson J, 2019). Products include Reflux Gourmet (refluxgourmet.com), Reflux Raft (refluxraft.com), Esophageal Guardian (www.lifeextension.com), and Gaviscon Advance (www.gaviscon.com).

Another study found that fenugreek fiber taken 30 minutes before meals significantly reduced heartburn symptoms based on symptom diaries and reduced medication use. The researchers report that the fenugreek fiber was similarly effective compared to H2 receptor antagonists (DiSilvestro RA, 2011).

Underhydration

The general rule is to drink about half as many ounces of water for each pound that you weigh.

Increasing water intake is of utmost importance for most people. Certain conditions including later stages of chronic kidney disease and congestive heart disease may require limiting water intake, but the general rule is to drink about half as many ounces of water for each pound that you weigh. For someone weighing 130 pounds this would be 2 quarts or 2 liters of water per day. There are apps available for smartphones that help you stay motivated and remember to drink water (ie Plant Nanny). For some people, trace minerals may be needed to make water work more effectively. There are many products on the market. Find one that doesn't have added sugar. An alternative is to add a pinch of

Redmond Real Salt to a glass of water. In addition, alkaline water (ie pH 8.8) has been shown to deactivate pepsin and buffer stomach acid, which may be quite helpful for acid reflux (Koufman JA, 2021).

CITATIONS

Yoon SL, Dietary Supplement and Complementary and Alternative Medicine Use Are Highly Prevalent in Patients with Gastrointestinal Disorders: Results from an Online Survey. J Diet Suppl. 2019;16(6):635-648. PMID: 29958032

Brown R et al, Effect of GutsyGum(tm), A Novel Gum, on Subjective Ratings of Gastro Esophageal Reflux Following A Refluxogenic Meal. J Diet Suppl. 2015 Jun;12(2):138-45. PMID: 25144853

Russell RI, Morgan RJ, Nelson LM, Studies on the protective effect of deglycyrrhinised liquorice against aspirin (ASA) and ASA plus bile acid-induced gastric mucosal damage, and ASA absorption in rats. Scand J Gastroenterol Suppl 1984;92:97-100. PMID: 6588541

Van Marle J, Aarsen PN, Lind A, van Weeren-Kramer J, Deglycyrrhizinised liquorice (DGL) and the renewal of rat stomach epithelium. Eur J Pharmacol. 1981 Jun 19;72(2-3):219-25. PMID: 7250207

Panahi Y et al, Efficacy and safety of Aloe vera syrup for the treatment of gastroesophageal reflux disease: a pilot randomized positive-controlled trial. J Tradit Chin Med, 35 (2015), pp. 632-636. PMID: 26742306

Yamanoi K, Nakayama J, Reduced αGlcNAc glycosylation on gastric gland mucin is a biomarker of malignant potential for gastric cancer, Barrett's adenocarcinoma, and pancreatic cancer. Histochem Cell Biol. 2018 Jun;149(6):569-575. PMID: 29658052

Kobayashi M, Lee H, Nakayama J, Fukudu M, Roles of gastric mucin-type O-glycans in the pathogenesis of Helicobacter pylori infection. Glycobiology. 2009 May;19(5):453-61. PMID: 19150806

Yamada S et al, Reduced gland mucin-specific O-glycan in gastric atrophy: A possible risk factor for differentiated-type adenocarcinoma of the stomach. J Gastroenterol Hepato. 2015 Oct;30(10):1478-84. PMID: 25967588

Ozbayoglu A et al, Effect of polaprezinc on experimental corrosive esophageal burns in rats. Dis Esophagus. 2017 Nov 1;30(11):1-6. PMID: 28881910

Choi HS et al, The effect of polaprezinc on gastric mucosal protection in rats with ethanol-induced gastric mucosal damage: comparison study with rebamipide. Life Sci. 2013 Jul 30;93(2-3):69-77. PMID: 23743168

Hewlings S, Kalman DA. Review of Zinc-L-Carnosine and Its Positive Effects on Oral Mucositis, Taste Disorders, and Gastrointestinal Disorders. Nutrients. 2020 Mar; 12(3): 665. PMID: 32121367

Hayashi H et al, Polaprezinc prevents oral mucositis in patients treated with high-dose chemotherapy followed by hematopoietic stem cell transplantation. Anticancer Res. 2014 Dec;34(12):7271-7. PMID: 25503160

Yanase K et al, Prevention of radiation esophagitis by polaprezinc (zinc L-carnosine) in patients with non-small cell lung cancer who received chemoradiotherapy. Int J Clin Exp Med. 2015; 8(9): 16215–16222. PMID: 26629136

Rao CV, Vijayakumar M. Effect of quercetin, flavonoids and α-tocopherol, an antioxidant vitamin on experimental reflux oesophagitis in rats. Eur J Pharmacol, 589 (2008), pp. 233-238. PMID: 18547560

Mahattanadul S et al, Effects of curcumin on reflux esophagitis in rats. J Nat Med. 2006 Jul;60(3):198-205. PMID: 29435885

Kwiecien S et al, Curcumin: A Potent Protectant against Esophageal and Gastric Disorders. Int J Mol Sci. 2019 Mar 24;20(6):1477. PMID: 30909623

Rawat N et al, Curcumin abrogates bile-induced NF-κB activity and DNA damage in vitro and suppresses NF-κB activity whilst promoting apoptosis in vivo, suggesting chemopreventative potential in Barrett's oesophagus. Clin Transl Oncol. 2012 Apr;14(4):302-11. PMID: 22484638

Konturek S.J., et al. Protective influence of melatonin against acute esophageal lesions involves prostaglandins, nitric oxide and sensory nerves. J. Physiol. Pharmacol. 2007;58:371–387. PMID: 17622703

Majka J et al, Melatonin in Prevention of the Sequence from Reflux Esophagitis to Barrett's Esophagus and Esophageal Adenocarcinoma: Experimental and Clinical Perspectives. Int J Mol Sci, 2018 Jul; 19(7): 2033. PMID: 30011784

Madalinski MH, Does a melatonin supplement alter the course of gastro-esophageal reflux disease? World J Gastrointest Pharmacol Ther. 2011 Dec 6;2(6):50-1. PMID: 22180850

Moraes TM et al, Healing actions of essential oils from Citrus aurantium and d-limonene in the gastric mucosa: the roles of VEGF, PCNA, and COX-2 in cell proliferation. J Med Food. 2013 Dec;16(12):1162-7. PMID: 24328705

Anandakumar P, Kamaraj S, Vanitha M. D-limonene: A multifunctional compound with potent therapeutic effects. J Food Biochem. 2021 Jan;45(1):e13566. PMID: 33289132

Kandil TS et al, The potential therapeutic effect of melatonin in gastro-esophageal reflux disease. BMC Gastroenterol. 2010; 10:7. PMID: 20082715

Pereira RdS, Regression of gastroesophageal reflux disease symptoms using dietary supplementation with melatonin, vitamins and amino acids: comparison with omeprazole. J Pinela Res. 2006 Oct;41(3):195-200. PMID: 16948779

Ortega MG, Agnese AM, Cabrera JL, Anticholinesterase activity in an alkaloid extract of Huperzia Saururus. Phytomedicine. 2004 Sept 20; 11(6):539-543. PMID: 15500266

Hägg M, Tibbling L, Franzén T. Esophageal dysphagia and reflux symptoms before and after oral IQoro training. World J Gastroenterol 2015; 21(24): 7558-7562. PMID: 26140003

Franzén T., Tibbling L., Hägg M. Oral neuromuscular training relieves hernia-related dysphagia and GERD symptoms as effectively in obese as in non-obese patients. Acta Oto-Laryngologica. Jan 2019;138(11):1-5. PMID: 30628501

Tam WC et al. Delivery of radiofrequency energy to the lower oesophageal sphincter and gastric cardia inhibits transient lower oesophageal sphincter relaxations and gastro-oesophageal reflux in patients with reflux disease. Gut. 2003 Apr;52(4):479-85. PMID: 12631654

Hu M-L et al, Effect of ginger on gastric motility and symptoms of functional dyspepsia. World H Gastroenterol. 2011 Jan 7; 17(1): 105–110. PMID 21218090

Wu K-L et al. Effects of ginger on gastric emptying and motility in healthy humans. Eur J Gastroenterol Hepatol. 2008 May;20(5):436-40. PMID: 21218090

Lazzini S et al, The effect of ginger (Zingiber officinalis) and artichoke (Cynara cardunculus) extract supplementation on gastric motility: a pilot randomized study in healthy volunteers. Eur Rev Med Pharmacol Sci 2016; 20 (1): 146-149. PMID: 26813467

Ghayur MN, Gilani AH, Pharmacological basis for the medicinal use of ginger in gastrointestinal disorders. Dig Dis Sci. 2005 Oct;50(10):1889-97. PMID: 16187193

Nikkhah Bodagh MN, Maleki I, Hekmatdoost A. Ginger in gastrointestinal disorders: A systematic review of clinical trials. Food Sci Nutr. 2018 Nov 5;7(1):96-108. PMID: 30680163

Saller R et al, Iberogast: a modern phytotherapeutic combined herbal drug for the treatment of functional disorders of the gastrointestinal tract (dyspepsia, irritable bowel syndrome)--from phytomedicine to "evidence based phytotherapy." A systematic review. Forsch Komplementarmed Klass Naturheilkd. 2002 Dec;9 Suppl 1:1-20. PMID: 12618546

Gerhardt F, Benesic A, Tillman HL, Rademacher S et al. Iberogast-Induced Acute Liver Failure-Reexposure and In Vitro Assay Support Causality, Am J Gastroenterol. 2019 Aug;114(8):1358-1359. PMID: 31246695

Chedid V et al. Herbal therapy is equivalent to rifaximin for the treatment of small intestinal bacterial overgrowth. Glob Adv Health Med. 2014 May;3(3):16-24. PMID: 24891990

Pimentel M et al, Methane, a gas produced by enteric bacteria, slows intestinal transit and augments small intestinal contractile activity. Am J Physiol Gastrointest Liver Physiol. 2006 Jun;290(6):G1089-95. PMID: 16293652

Ojetti V et al, Effect of Lactobacillus reuteri (DSM 17938) on methane production in patients affected by functional constipation: a retrospective study. Eur Rev Med Pharmacol Sci. 2017 Apr;21(7):1702-1708. PMID: 28429333

Brown K, Scott-Hoy B, Jennings LJ. Response of irritable bowel syndrome with constipation patients administered a combined quebracho/conker tree/M. balsamea Willd extract. World J Gastrointest Pharm Ther. 2016 Aug 6;7(3):463-468. PMID 27602249

Wilkinson J et al. Randomized clinical trial: a double-blind, placebo-controlled study to assess the clinical efficacy and safety of alginate-antacid (Gaviscon Double Action) chewable tablets in patients with gastro-oesophageal reflux disease. Eur J Gastroenterol Hepatol. 2019 Jan;31(1):86-93. PMID: 30272584

DiSilvestro RA, Verbruggen MA, Offutt EJ, Anti-heartburn effects of a fenugreek fiber product. Phytother Res. 2011 Jan;25(1):88-91. PMID: 20623611

Koufman JA, Johnston N. Potential benefits of pH 8.8 alkaline drinking water as an adjunct in the treatment of reflux disease. Ann Otol Rhinol Laryngol. 2012 Jul;121(7):431-4. PMID: 22844861

ELEVEN

Your Brain May Be Sabotaging Your Digestion

by Kayle Sandberg-Lewis, LMT, MA, BCN-Fellow

We evolved to be real brainiacs,
But our brains may misread what we track.
Our guts feel on fire
And life seems quite dire,
'Til we remedy what's out of whack.

We evolved to have brains big and strong,
But sometimes the base gets things wrong.
We see danger where it's not
Or just react to a thought,
And our guts play some painful ping-pong.

KEY QUESTIONS

What role does the brain play in digestive health?

What is chronic hyperventilation, and how may it affect digestion?

How might I learn to fool my brain into thinking the world is a safe place?

THE ORIENTATION RESPONSE

Let's pretend we're furry little mammals, munching on grubs somewhere out on the veld approximately 178 million years ago. Suddenly, we hear a sharp snap. Immediately we stop eating, jerk our heads up, hold our breath and listen in what scientists now call the orientation response. [Back then we just called it, "What was THAT?"] If the noise came from a predator, we needed to run away. If it was one of our family members—clumsy Cousin Clarence, for example—we probably shuddered for a few moments, sighed, and got back to eating.

When there was a real danger, those of us who did not respond fast enough were probably a tasty snack for some predator while those among us who had an effective "orientation response" were more apt to run away, live through the ordeal and reproduce, passing on our superior neurological reflexes to our offspring.

Over the years, this response became more and more refined—"hard wired" into each new generation. So here we are in the 21st century with three and a half trillion generations of practice. We're so good at this response, it can be elicited by the phone ringing, someone tapping us on the shoulder, someone mentioning "taxes" or any other of an endless list of triggers.

The Brainstem and Autonomic Nervous System

It turns out that all that evolution left one little part of our brain in charge of keeping us alive—the brainstem. Also known as the reptilian brain because even reptiles have them, the brainstem is situated like a clenched fist at the top of the spinal cord. All the rest of your magnificent brain grew above and beyond it, including the parts that speak, reason and love. The brainstem has no language skills. You cannot take it to therapy.

Housed in the brainstem is the autonomic nervous system (ANS). As the name suggests, it is a nervous system for the "automatic" functions of the body—because you really don't want to have to <u>think</u> about breathing and making your heart beat while doing the dishes or walking the dog. Sleeping would be impossible if one had to consciously dictate each inhalation/exhalation cycle, let alone the gyrations of the migrating motor complex, the cleansing cycle our intestines go through during sleep.

The brainstem does this for you, closely monitoring your breathing, cardiac activity, and other vital functions of your body when both awake and asleep. It behaves somewhat like a meter reader—paying attention to all sorts of "readings" in your system and looking for things to go wonky. It attends to your hydration level, your sugar levels, how much oxygen you have and many, many more life sustaining processes. But without language skills, it is not able to gently inform you of a problem. It can't calmly say to you, "You are becoming dehydrated. Better pour yourself a glass of

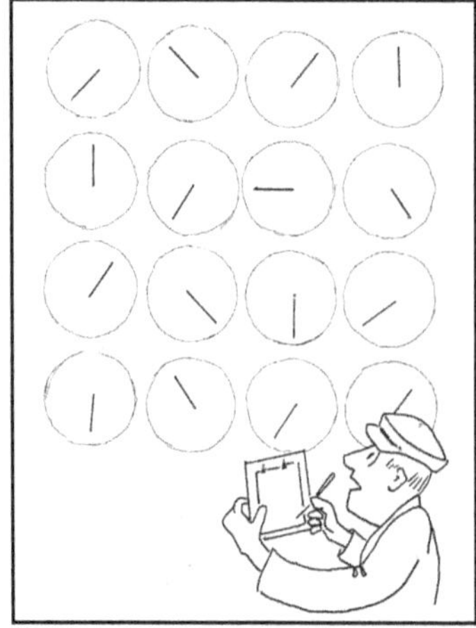

Autonomic Nervous System —the meter reader in the brain.

Fig. 11.1. Imagining the brainstem as a meter reader.

water." All it knows how to do is set off alarms. So, the alarm for dehydration often goes off at about 3AM. You are suddenly wide awake, but you don't know why. Instead of the brainstem directing you to reach for water, the verbal part of your brain is probably going to seize upon events or thoughts that have absolutely nothing to do with dehydration and you lie awake, ruminating about the guy who cut you off in traffic or what you should have said to that overbearing customer.

Sympathetic Nervous System

It is likely you already know the branch of the autonomic nervous system that woke you by its nickname, "fight or flight". Its proper name is sympathetic nervous system (SNS), and it is associated with high arousal. "Sympathetic" sounds nice, right? It is based on the idea that the parts of the body are connected —in sympathy—with each other. The SNS is, essentially, looking for trouble because it and its counterpart, the parasympathetic nervous system (PNS), are tasked with keeping you alive. The SNS is on alert to mobilize your reserves to deal with mortal threats. The problem is that if you spend too much time in sympathetic dominance, you will develop anxiety and stress-related disorders such as hypertension, migraines, and digestive disorders.

Parasympathetic Nervous System

The other branch of the autonomic nervous system, the parasympathetic, has a nickname too, although it is not as well known. It is "rest and digest" and is associated with lower arousal and building the body's reserves. While we need both aspects of the autonomic system, it makes sense that the majority of our time is best spent in parasympathetic dominance.

You have probably experienced a noticeable shift in your own balance between sympathetic and parasympathetic dominance many times. Too much caffeine, too little sleep, and/or low blood sugar and we are more apt to startle easily, not think clearly, or lash out at someone. On the other hand, deep rest can result in a sense of resilience and increased capacity to face challenges.

Reduce the Effects of Stressors

In my vision of the metaphorical meters our brain stem reads, the needle represents the stressor and can move to reflect the immediacy of an issue.

The SNS is on alert to mobilize your reserves to deal with mortal threats.

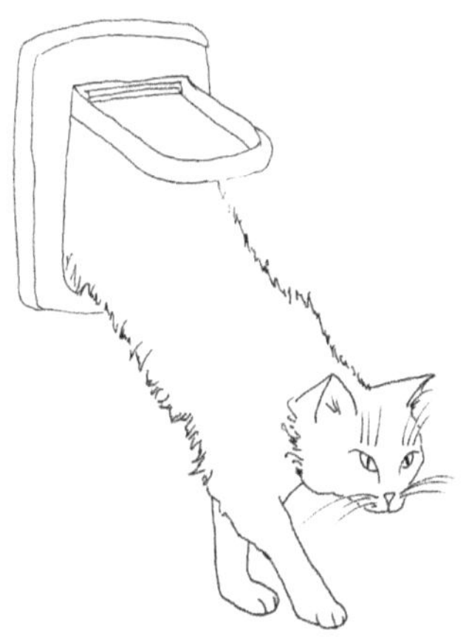

Fig. 11.2. The autonomic nervous system is a lot like a cat door.

When considering the balance between parasympathetic and sympathetic dominance, it may help to think of a cat door. While it swings both in and out, it cannot work in both directions at the same time.

When the brainstem assumes a situation is dangerous, "rest and digest" turns off while the body's reserves are mobilized to preserve life.

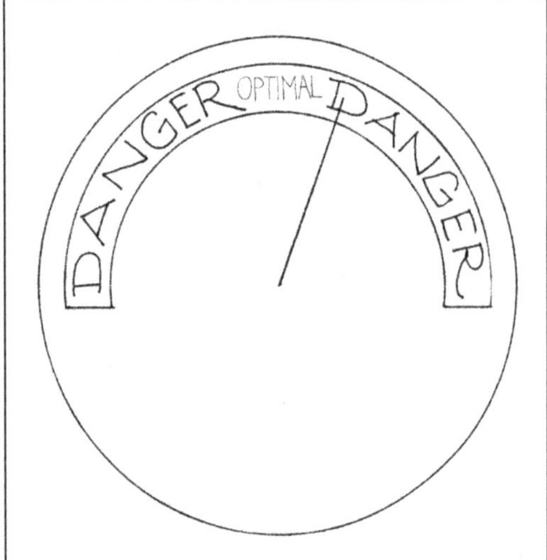

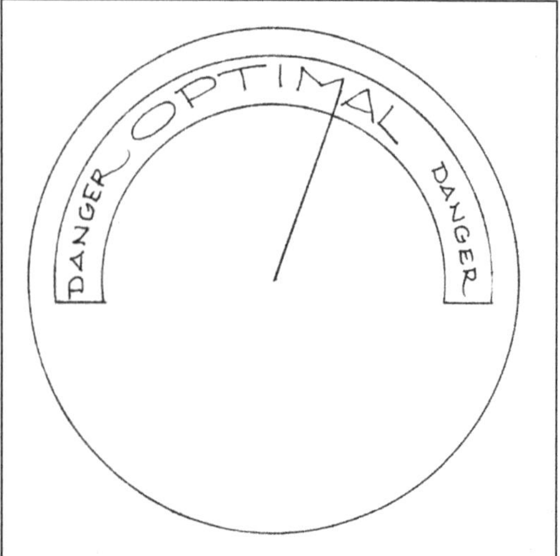

Fig. 11.3. Representation of someone easily triggered into sympathetic dominance.

Fig. 11.4. Representation of someone who has expanded her capacity to deal with stress.

In the above illustrations, however, the needle is in the same location on the meters, but the "optimal" zone (parasympathetic dominance) changes. The left meter represents an individual who has low reserves and is easily triggered into sympathetic dominance. The right meter represents someone who has worked to expand their psychophysiological capacity to deal with stress.

Psychophysiology: The relationship between signals from the body and mental/emotional processes.

While you cannot talk your brainstem into being calm and parasympathetically dominant—at least not easily—you can *fool* your brainstem into thinking the world is a safe place where you can live in relative peace. The beauty of this subterfuge is, essentially, an expansion of the "optimal" zone on the meter—more parasympathetic dominance—which generally means better sleep, more efficient digestion, and healthier interactions with others. You may call this stress management. Scientists call it "cultivated low arousal".

Cultivating Low Arousal

The brainstem sets off alarms when it perceives something to be life threatening—no matter whether that perception is accurate. Yet, there are ways to turn off the alarms and, even better, there are ways to keep them from setting off in the first place. Let's start at the <u>end</u> of our stress response.

Cultivated Low Arousal: Reducing anxiety by fooling your brain into believing that the world is safe.

Harking back to the early mammals on the veld when our pursuit of a meal was interrupted by the sudden snapping of a twig, something that could easily indicate an approaching predator, we held our breath, jerked our heads back and swiveled our ears around to ascertain more information. If we figured out there was no immediate danger, we probably shuddered, sighed, and got back to eating.

What is the shuddering/sighing about?

The stress response sets in motion a huge cascade of physiological/biochemical responses, preparing the body to run for its life or to fight. All systems are affected. Cardiovascular, hormonal, neurological, emotional, metabolic, pulmonary, gastrointestinal systems are shifted from low arousal to high arousal and put on red alert—the needle goes into the "danger zone". Even our skin changes! Energy is mobilized. What happens to all that energy if it is unnecessary or disproportionate to the situation? How do all those reactions get "undone"?

Keep in mind that the brainstem

(1) has not caught up with the modern world. It may interpret something like the phone ringing or a snarky comment on Facebook as a mortal threat. (This happens not because of the words in the post but because of your emotional reaction. The brainstem eavesdrops on your affect and takes its cues accordingly.)

(2) has no language skills—you can't simply say, "Oh sweet, overly reactive Brainstem, it was a false alarm. We are safe" and expect it to respond properly. You must SHOW it you are safe. But how?

RELEASING THE STRESS RESPONSE

As the American singer-songwriter Taylor Swift advises, SHAKE IT OFF.

Robert Sapolsky's *Why Zebras Don't Get Ulcers*, first published in 1994, is a detailed account of what unprocessed stress does to the human body and mind. (The title gives a hint that zebras have a better coping mechanism than many humans.) In 1997, Peter Levine published his revolutionary book, *Waking the Tiger: Healing Trauma*. Both Sapolsky and Levine looked to the natural world for insight on how to deal with the stress response. It turns out the shuddering/sighing behavior is <u>therapeutic</u>. It is a universal response among animals when they escape from their predators. Through this physical response, the body shifts out of "danger" and communicates to the brainstem all is safe.

What if there isn't a major event that has a clear end but

instead a chronic stressor like an irritating co-worker or recurring problem with transportation? Maybe the landlord hasn't addressed a faulty furnace. Your brainstem may still send signals through your system that there is constant danger because it just doesn't "get" nuance. Even more onerous are the day-to-day grinding indignities due to systemic racial and/or sexual discrimination. Unlike a confrontation with a clear end, you are not apt to go through the shudder/sigh release automatically because the stressor is ongoing.

I mentioned earlier the tactic of fooling your brainstem into thinking the world is a safe place. We can do that by <u>behaving</u> as though we are safe, even though the more evolved parts of our brains are aware of the existence of hazards in the world. We just need to keep that information from affecting our brainstems. There are many cues the brainstem is "reading" to figure out how to respond. If your <u>behavior</u> is convincing, the brainstem will turn off the alarms. "Things must be OK if she's doing THAT."

To be effective, you can retrain yourself to release the pent-up energy as soon as you are able. In *Walking Your Blues Away*, (2006), Thom Hartmann makes an excellent case for processing emotions through swinging the arms in an alternate rhythm to the legs (also called "cross crawl") while walking. Emily Nagoski and Amelia Nagoski, *Burnout* (2020), stress the need to "complete the stress cycle" through running, dancing, or other vigorous physical activities.

By releasing the stress response, you can save yourself from accumulating the effects chronic stress has on your body. *Stress and trauma are experienced physiologically and must be released physically.* No matter what your physical abilities, there are exercises that help this process. [Whatever exercise you choose, doing it long enough to sweat is generally even more helpful.]

Now that we know how to disperse the effects of the stress response after it has occurred—shuddering and sighing, [Sighing—there is that exhalation again!] let's talk about how our breathing patterns can TRIGGER the stress response and keep us on edge.

HOW BREATHING PATTERNS TRIGGER THE STRESS RESPONSE

Remember that veld where we were gathering grubs a few millennia ago? We heard the twig snap, jerked our heads back and

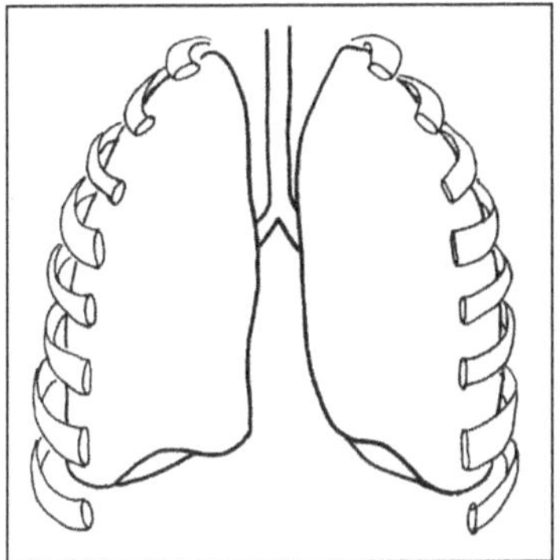

Fig. 11.5 The lungs occupy most of the thoracic cavity.

The left lung has a little cave where the heart sits and does its work. The tops of the lungs rest just behind your collarbones and the bases of the lungs are down there at the bottom of your ribcage, resting atop the diaphragm.

The lungs are extraordinarily delicate and need all the bones of the ribcage to help prevent bruising or punctures from our day-to-day activities.

stopped breathing—all at once. Breathing can be noisy and holding the breath can give us a moment to determine the presence and direction of potential harm. It is meant to be momentary and then we either run like crazy or resume what we were doing after sighing and shuddering.

What if we resume what we were doing but keep breathing shallowly? Or worse, don't breathe much at all?

While the brainstem is "listening in" on what we do and how we react, it is making assumptions—generally negative—about the danger we are facing. This can trigger and then maintain a level of anxiety that makes life less enjoyable than it might otherwise be. If we do not shudder and sigh, and resume breathing but do so shallowly—so the breath enters only the upper parts of our lungs—we are telling the eavesdropping brainstem that the threat continues. Plus, because the lungs are shaped the way they are, we are inhaling less air when we breathe shallowly, causing us to breathe more rapidly to come close to the gas exchange required to keep us alive.

DISORDERED BREATHING CAN SEEM "NORMAL"

There are three names for this rapid breathing/breath holding pattern: Breathing Pattern Disorders, Chronic Hyperventilation, and Over Breathing. Most of us are familiar with "hyperventilation". It can be caused by several organic conditions such as diabetic ketoacidosis or pregnancy, but it is exceedingly rare. Actual hyperventilation, by definition, is breathing in excess of 22 breaths per minute, and makes up only 1% of the cases. It is an acute condition. The remaining 99% of the cases are chronic.

Chronic hyperventilation can feel "normal", even when interspersed with breath holding. At 18 to 20 breaths per minute, it is just enough slower that people can become accustomed to it. It is important to note we are talking about a resting state. How rapidly you breathe should be dependent on your physical activity. Exerting yourself physically is going to require more frequent gas exchange than when at rest. Therefore, the definition of chronic hyperventilation stipulates "breathing in excess of metabolic requirements". You SHOULD breathe more frequently when climbing a mountain or salsa dancing than when sitting in a recliner.

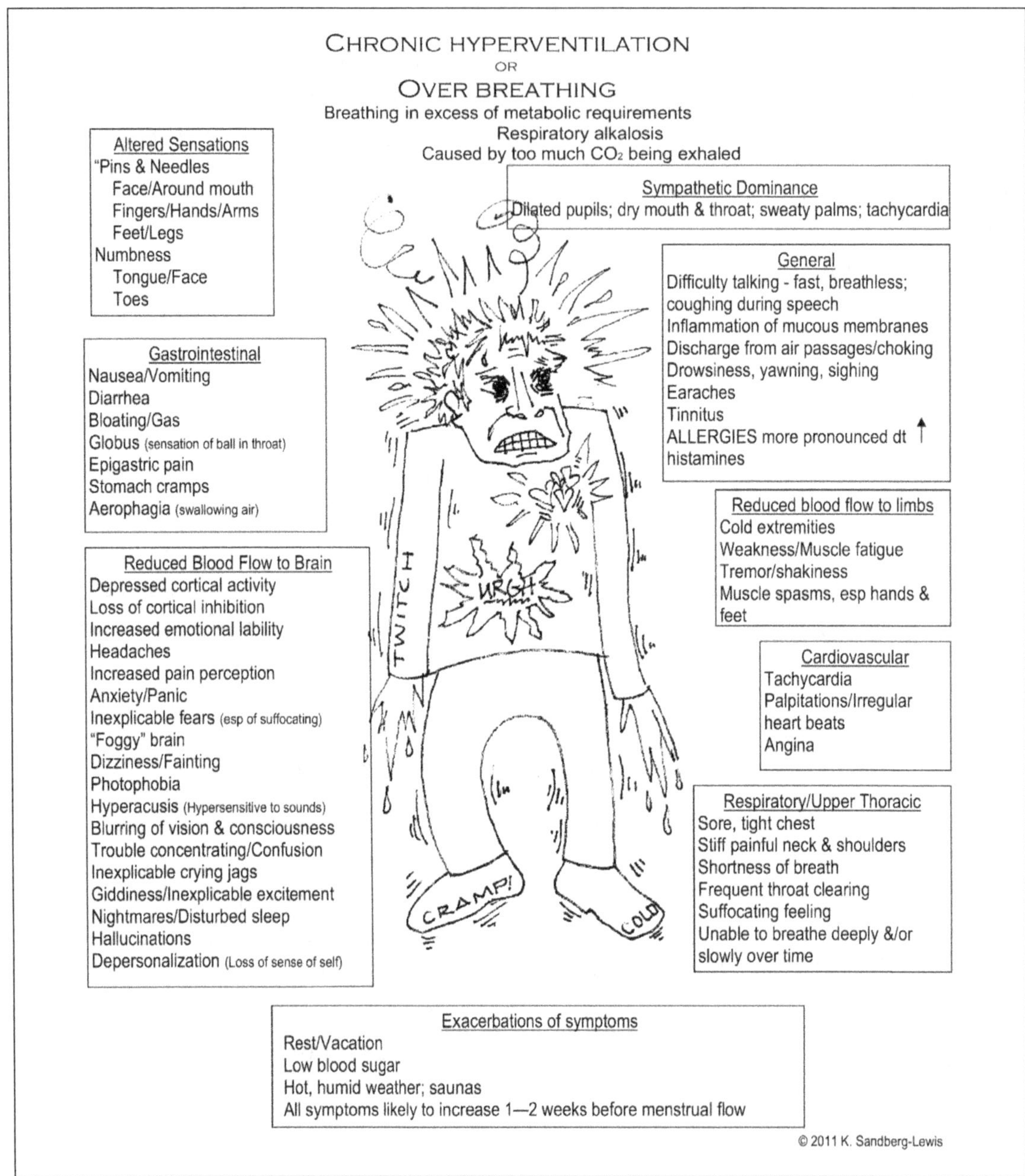

Fig. 11.6. The many effects of chronic hyperventilation or overbreathing.

Take a look at the drawing above of the fellow I call a truly miserable man. Clustered around him are the many issues triggered by over breathing.

EXERCISES TO CHANGE YOUR BREATHING PATTERNS

So now you have an idea of what chronic hyperventilation can cause, but how do you change your breathing patterns? I will be the first to admit it is NOT easy. You probably learned maladaptive breathing rather early in life and since breathing is governed primarily by the autonomic nervous system, it goes unobserved for the most part. Trying to change something that engrained will not happen quickly.

EXERCISES

Lungs do not breathe by themselves. They rely on surrounding muscles to create changes in pressure on the lungs. When the muscles pull away, the air pressure in the lungs drops to less than the air pressure in the room —air leaves the room and enters the lungs. When the muscles press in, the air pressure in the lungs increases, becoming greater than the pressure in the room and the lungs exhale.

The primary and ideal muscle for this pushing and pulling is the diaphragm. Unfortunately, with shallow breathing, the muscles of the neck and shoulders are recruited instead of the diaphram which means the neck and shoulder muscles are doing "pullups" from 18–20 times per minute. No wonder your neck and shoulders are so sore!

(1) Pick three "prompts" or "cues"—my suggestions are doorknobs, faucets, and light switches because they occur throughout most days and are transitional in nature—going from one room to another; going from dry to wet; going from dark to light or vice versa.

As you reach out, take a slow breath in, counting to 4 or so. You will become more comfortable with longer inhalations the more often you do the exercise.

Hold your breath for a count of two.

Purse your lips and slowly exhale through them as you count backwards from 8 to 1. (However long it took to inhale, double that time for exhaling.) Then go about your day until you encounter the next cue.

If you do this throughout the day, you will become more aware of your breathing patterns and more likely to catch yourself when you either hold your breath or breathe shallowly.

(2) Practice diaphragmatic breathing *to the best of your ability*.

While sitting or standing, place your hands at your sides, touching the base of your ribcage. As you inhale, your ribcage should move outwards. This is an indication that your diaphragm has engaged, and you are breathing into the lowest lobes of your lungs.

Breathe in slowly through your nose, which cleans the air and adjusts the air temperature before it reaches those oh so delicate lungs. The last aspect of your body to expand should be the upper chest. Exhale slowly through your nose or pursed lips. When breathing in this manner, a full cycle of breaths will occur six to eight times per minute, just the right speed to soothe the vagus nerve.

Please note: If you have been doing the shallow breathing throughout your life, your body, in its wisdom, has probably turned to a compensatory mechanism called the Bohr effect that will make slow diaphragmatic breathing very difficult. You may get dizzy, angry, antsy, see spots. There are many possible responses because you are suddenly flooding your system with much more oxygen than it is accustomed to dealing with. If after a few minutes, you feel uncomfortable doing slow, deep breathing, return to just doing the type of breathing in exercise 1 above. It will, over time, uncouple the Bohr effect and allow you to do the deep, soothing diaphragmatic breathing you deserve.

BREATHE WITH THE DIAPHRAGM AND LOWER ANXIETY

Why is breathing with the diaphragm so important in lowering anxiety? The diaphragm is innervated by the tenth cranial nerve (CN X) or vagus nerve which is both a motor nerve (it tells several organs what to do) AND a sensory nerve—it tells the brain what those organs are doing. When it is not engaged and the breathing is shallow, and therefore rapid, the brainstem gets the message and interprets it as DANGER. When the diaphragm is moving smoothly and slowly, the brainstem believes all's right with the world. After all, how else could one breathe so peacefully?

NOT CHEWING MAY BE YOUR UNDOING (CHAPTER ONE LIMERICK)

We've discussed the role of the vagus nerve—both a motor and sensory nerve that innervates several organs including the lungs—in soothing the brainstem when we simply slow our breath to around 6 – 8 breaths per minute (unless we have accommodated less functional breathing with the Bohr effect).

Another cranial nerve, the trigeminal nerve, or CN V, also performs both motor and sensory functions. It innervates the muscles of the mouth, allowing us to chew and swallow AND, in its sensory capacity, takes information back to the brainstem.

How do you suppose the brainstem interprets the information from the trigeminal nerve when a person bolts food on the run? Eats distractedly while driving? Takes a bite and then swigs a drink to wash it down? Danger! Even eating quickly while seated at the table can tell the already "nervous" brainstem to stay in the danger zone.

CHEW YOUR FOOD

Thoroughly chewing your food not only breaks it down mechanically; it also starts the chemical breakdown of the food as the enzymes in your saliva saturate each morsel. Chew each bite of solid food until it is liquified. Do this without adding water or other beverages. Just chew. Thoroughly breaking down the fibers of food in the mouth makes the stomach's job much easier.

The most common response I have received when I coach people on chewing is, "But that is so BORING!" It doesn't have to be.

Many belief systems hold that the body is the temple of the soul. Try that idea on while planning your dining experience.

Some people have difficulty engaging their diaphragms, usually because of an abdominal injury or scar tissue from surgery. In such situations, I recommend finding a body worker who is versed in Structural Integration or Myofascial Release.

The day we were born, the first thing we did was inhale—we became "inspired". When we die, the last thing we do is exhale and we "expire". Most of us would prefer our expiration date come later rather than sooner. Proper breathing can help.

Aim for making your meals a sacred time when you slow down and care for the temple. Light candles or just lower the lights. Play soothing music. If you don't have fresh flowers, a picture of flowers can help your system slow down. You might try putting down your fork or spoon while chewing, folding your hands in your lap. Conversation about positive issues is helpful. It is common for people who live alone to resist this suggestion, saying it is hard enough to plan the food and fix it for one person let alone to create a "dining experience", but those who have reported back after trying it have told me it has transformed their mealtimes into something they look forward to.

If you still complain that focusing on chewing is just too tedious, I'm not going to argue with you. I just ask you to think of your antsy little brainstem, lulled into a peaceful rest by that slow, rhythmic chewing.

SUFFICIENT WATER IS VITAL FOR YOUR GOOD HEALTH

Back to our "meter reader". It notes levels of vital elements for physiological functioning and sets off alarms when the monitored element goes "out of bounds". It does this because your brainstem perceives your life to be in danger. Unfortunately, because of the brainstem's nonverbal nature, it can't tell you what is out of whack.

You have undoubtedly heard the phrase "water is life." That is shorthand for "without water, life's many processes will grind to a desiccated and tragic halt; without enough water, life is at risk of becoming a congested, clogged mess." The same holds true for your body—water is vital for good health from cognition to cardiac function, from renal to respiratory activity, and more.

Without enough pure, clean water, your body simply cannot work efficiently. In fact, lack of water will set off that meter reader in your brainstem and will cause a general sense of anxiety and may wake you in the middle of the night, usually between 1 and 3 am. Most people interpret their awakening as a need to go to the bathroom, but it is not uncommon for these same people to report they void very little urine during their trip(s) to the loo. And generally, these same people, upon getting back in bed, have a heck of a time returning to sleep.

Clients often assure me they get enough water because they drink lots of coffee, tea, and other beverages. Here's the problem:

Wet does not equal water. These drinks, especially those containing caffeine or alcohol, are dehydrating, causing the body to lose water, and they are adding "nutrients" that must be metabolized before any water that is present can be used. It is recommended that for each cup of non-water a cup of pure water be consumed.

Clients express fear that drinking more water than they already do will further interrupt their sleep.

Being adequately hydrated tends to improve sleep simply because the "dehydration alarm" will not go off. Yes, you may need to get up once to void your bladder, but you will probably find it much easier to return to sleep.

I understand when people tell me they don't like to drink water. I grew up in a town that heavily chlorinated its reservoir and a glass of water from the tap smelled and tasted like the municipal pool. It was metallic and sometimes it made my teeth hurt or my throat sore. Consequently, I rarely drank plain water. I was also ill a lot as a child.

Depending on where you live, you may have a similar experience—perhaps your tap yields brackish water or some other contaminant that causes you to avoid hydrating. In the US, municipalities tend to oversee water quality with standards set by states and, more often, the federal government's Environmental Protection Agency (EPA). Unfortunately, oversight can be lax, and lately some regulations have been relaxed rather than strengthened. [According to Deanna DeLong in *Drink Water for Life, Your Journey to Better Health*, over 2,100 contaminants have been identified in US drinking water, but the EPA regulates only 89.]

What I Recommend

1. If your water source is less than optimal, find a source of pure water, whether by putting a filter on your kitchen sink or a sourcing at a local grocery.

2. Figure out how much water you should consume in a day. The formula is simple: Divide your total body weight (in pounds) by two and drink that many ounces of pure water. (e.g., A half ounce per pound. If you weigh 150 pounds, drink 75 ounces.) First thing in the morning, fill either glass or stainless-steel bottles with the total amount of water you should imbibe and place them somewhere

Please avoid plastic containers. The phthalates or plasticizers in the containers leach into the water and are carried into our bodies where they act as endocrine disruptors.

conspicuous such as your kitchen counter. I make this suggestion because we tend to inadvertently "cheat"—telling ourselves we refilled a bottle two or three times when we did not. To have the bottles staring at me tends to hold me accountable.

DRINK MORE WATER

3. If you are physically active, increase the amount of water to 2/3 ounce per pound to help replace what you lose through sweat and breathing harder. If the weather is particularly hot and you are exercising, increase your water intake to about a cup every quarter hour while active.

4. Start your day with a large glass of water before you eat or drink anything else.

5. Drink a glass of water about a half hour before meals.

6. Drink another large glass of water about an hour or so after a meal.

What has proven fascinating about following this protocol is the consistent reports I receive. At first people report increased urge to urinate and then, as their bodies acclimate to the increased level of water, they need fewer trips to the loo. Also, people who had insisted they did not experience thirst reported starting to recognize a craving for water. Generally, sleep improves, anxiety as well as body aches are reduced, bowel function improves, and people report they experience less joint pain and an improved complexion.

FOOLING YOUR BRAINSTEM LOWERS ANXIETY

My goal is to help you understand how much influence you have over the brainstem where arousal-anxiety lives. You do not need to be a victim of your anxiety. Instead, you can change your behaviors to convince your brainstem the world is a safe place.

The brainstem is reading the "meters" in your system—evaluating whether you are safe and setting off alarms when it perceives danger, even if there is no real threat. The "meters" we have focused on have to do with life sustaining issues such as hydration and respiration—issues you can affect by changing your behavior. We also talked about mindfully chewing your food in order to send the message to your brainstem that you are safe.

But what happens when you forget and revert to old behaviors?

Maybe you catch yourself breathing shallowly, bolting your food and/or not drinking the water you know you need. How do you respond when you notice?

We talked about shuddering or otherwise physically working out the pent-up tension. What we have not yet addressed is our emotional response. What do you say to yourself when you notice your lapse? Is it some version of, "I'll never get this right"? Or "I'm so stupid"? Or "I'll never be healthy if I can't do this."?

Your self-talk is the key to your self-care.

To truly practice self-care, you must treat yourself with loving kindness. Depending on your upbringing, this may be the hardest shift of all. We often absorb messages from our childhood about performance and our capacity to do the "right" thing. We may have set unattainable standards for ourselves and may spend time berating ourselves for not meeting criteria.

Perhaps you are a perfectionist.

I'm not a diagnostician but I AM a recovering perfectionist and I have come to believe perfectionism is at the root of most stress related disorders. Many of my clients try to argue with me about this. Their position, invariably, is that a deep desire to do things "right" can't possibly be bad. Perfectionism, however, is never that simple and altruistic. I think of it as a mis-guided religion—a belief that things can be perfect and that if we can attain that, we can—at least for a moment—justify our existence.

Perfectionism, at its core, is a need for control. Granted, a desire to control variables and having an eye for details is a good thing when it comes to flying a plane or performing brain surgery, but those same "skills" aren't well transferred to parenting, maintaining friendships, or nurturing your own wellbeing.

There is a language of perfectionism—it's full of imperatives: "Must!" "Should!" "Always!" "NEVER!" These words are emotionally loaded and can trigger your brainstem to set off the alarms we're trying to avoid. Why?

While the brainstem doesn't have language skills to express itself and cannot be taken to therapy, it does listen to the emotional tone of self-talk. So, when you berate yourself for "failing",

Being angry with yourself is counterproductive.

the brainstem is eavesdropping and sensing that YOU think you have blundered—which it interprets as dangerous and a threat to your survival. (Remember, the brainstem is still living in the world of predators where mistakes are fatal.)

As I said, this is a topic I know all too intimately and I am aware that cheery self-talk is unlikely to feel appropriate, let alone help. "You're the greatest!" is not going to work in dissuading a perfectionist.

Create new habits starting with, "Thanks for the reminder."

What I have found to be helpful is a more neutral response. Notice you are holding your breath or breathing shallowly? Try saying, "Thanks for the reminder," and then practice your slow breathing with even slower exhalations. Realize you've gulped your food? "Thanks for the reminder," and slow your chewing so the next bite is liquid before you swallow it. I believe "Thanks for the reminder" works because it takes the pressure off. It gives us another chance to do what needs to be done. The more frequently we lovingly correct our course, the more likely it will become a new default behavior. A new habit.

We are in the business of repair. With practice and loving kindness toward yourself, you can do this.

CITATIONS

Hartmann, T. (2006). Walking Your Blues Away: How to Heal the Mind and Create Emotional Well-Being (Second Printing). Park Street Press.

How to calculate how much water you should drink | University of Missouri System. (n.d.). https://www.umsystem.edu/totalrewards/wellness/how-to-calculate-how-much-water-you-should-drink

Levine, P. A., & Frederick, A. (1997). Waking the Tiger: Healing Trauma North Atlantic Books.

Nagoski, E., & Nagoski, A. (2020). Burnout: The Secret to Unlocking the Stress Cycle. Ballantine Books.

Sapolsky, R. M. (2004). Why Zebras Don't Get Ulcers, (3rd edition). Holt Paperbacks.

Yamada, Y., Zhang, X., Henderson, M. E. T., & Sagayama, H. (2022). Variation in human water turnover associated with environmental and lifestyle factors. Science, 378(6622), 909–915. https://doi.org/10.1126/science.abm8668

TWELVE

Hiatal Hernia and Hiatal Hernia Syndrome

The respiratory diaphragm divides
The thorax from its undersides.
When the two intermix,
It's important to fix,
The resultant hernia that slides.

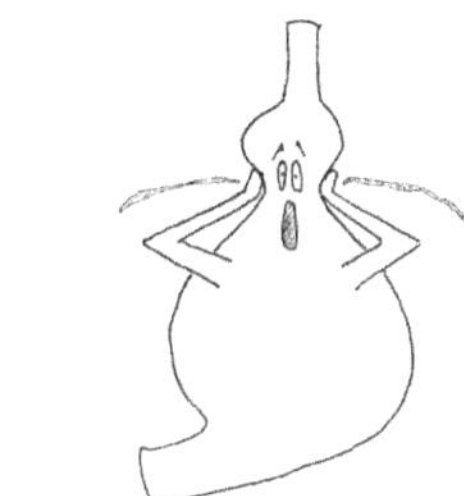

Fig 12.1. With apologies to Edvard Munch.

Glossary

thoracic—referring to the chest

abdominal—referring to the abdomen or belly

hypermobility syndrome—a genetic condition that involves extreme joint and tissue flexibility which can cause joint injuries, digestive disorders and other effects.

tortuous—having many twists and turns

redundant—excessively long as in redundant colon

KEY QUESTIONS

Is there a difference between a hiatal hernia and the hiatal hernia syndrome?

What is a sliding hiatal hernia?

What is the connection between reflux and hiatal hernias?

Anatomy of a Hiatal Hernia

Anatomy textbooks show the internal organs placed just so. While organs tend to be located "where they belong" most of the time, there can be surprises. Fig.12.2. illustrates the typical, expected location of the abdominal organs, which are below the diaphragm. The thoracic area, above the diaphragm, contains the heart and lungs. As I noted, this is not accurate for every individual. Some of us have "alternate anatomy" such as a sliding hiatal hernia which can

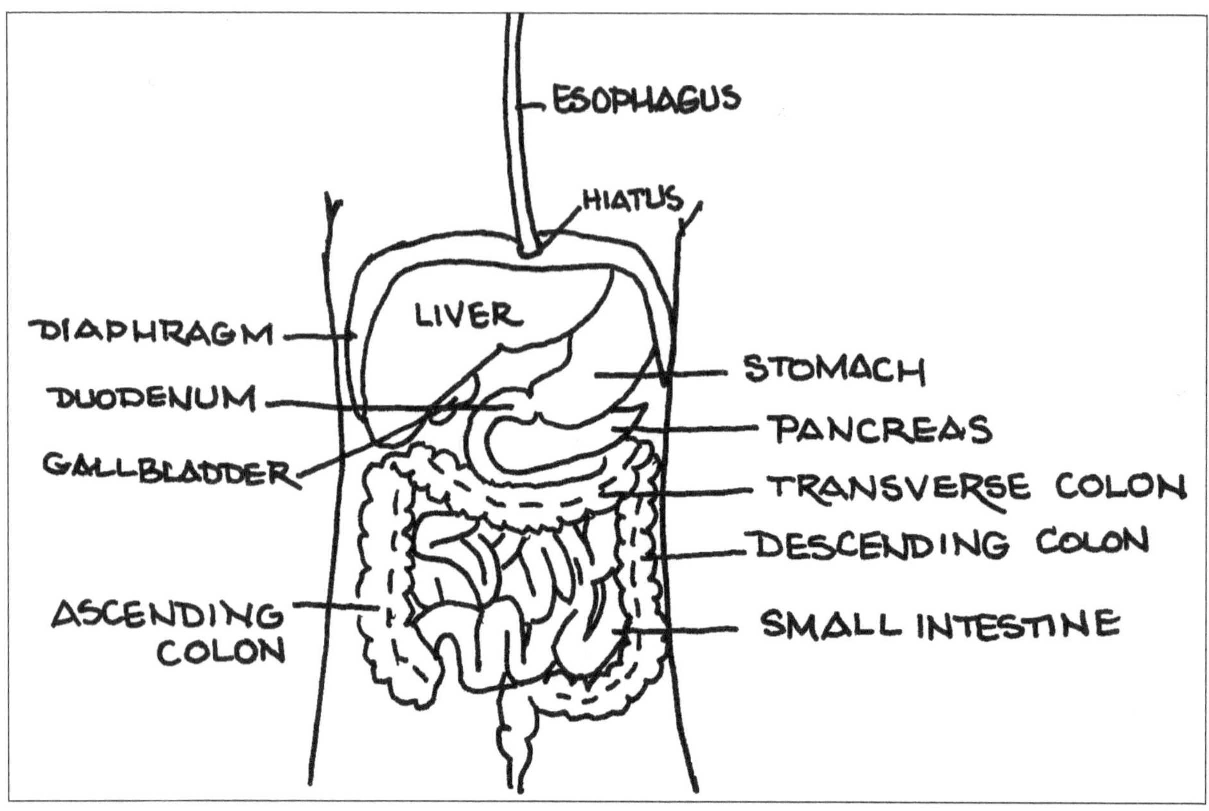

Fig. 12.2. Typical abdominal anatomy.

intermittently slide the upper portion of the stomach through the hiatus of the diaphragm into the thorax. A sliding hiatal hernia can move the upper stomach two or more centimeters into the chest. As discussed in chapter two, the LES needs the support of the diaphragm to keep the stomach contents from refluxing. When a portion of the stomach breeches the diaphragm, the LES is much less effective. The small portion of the stomach above the diaphragm is also a reservoir for stomach acid, increasing the acid pocket (Menezes MA, 2017).

A sliding hiatal hernia can move the upper stomach two or more centimeters into the chest.

Those with hypermobility syndromes are especially prone to sliding hiatal hernia.

The stomach is typically tucked up underneath the left dome of the respiratory diaphragm. According to the 2006 edition of the Merck Manual, up to 40 percent of Americans have a sliding hiatal hernia (Berkow R, 2006). The prevalence increases to 60% in senior citizens (Smith AB, 1999). It can travel back and forth between the abdomen and the chest. Those with **hypermobility syndromes** are especially prone to sliding hiatal hernia (Castori M et al, 2015). A rare form of hiatal hernia is called paraesophageal hernia, which is not the topic of this chapter.

Another common example of alternate anatomy is a **tortuous, redundant** colon, with the normally upside-down U shape of the large intestine altered. It is longer than usual, exhibiting many extra folds, bends and turns. This anatomically abnormal shape may be the case in both people who have suffered from long-term states of constipation and those with lax collagen as found in hypermobility syndromes.

Fig. 12.3. shows the difference between the normal stomach position on the left, and a sliding hiatal hernia on the right.

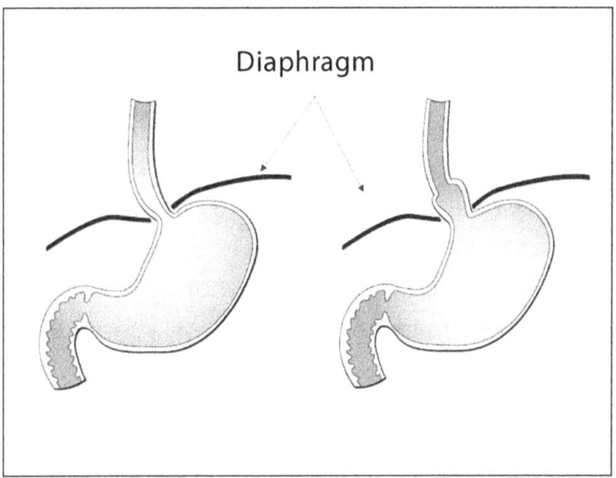

Fig 12.3. Normal stomach position on left, and a sliding hiatal hernia on the right.

As illustrated above, the bulge of the upper stomach pushes the LES above the diaphragm, and into the chest. This often weakens the LES and allows GERD to occur.

By design, the walls of all the digestive organs, from the esophagus down to the anus, are muscular tubes designed to move food downward. If everything is moving down, why would the stomach move up?

CAUSES OF SLIDING HIATAL HERNIA

PRESSURE DIFFERENTIAL BETWEEN THE ABDOMEN AND CHEST

The respiratory diaphragm divides the trunk of the body into the chest and the abdomen. Everything above is **thoracic**, and everything below is **abdominal**. A sliding hiatal hernia, and therefore reflux, can occur when increases in intra-abdominal pressure, meaning pressure levels located below the diaphragm, overpower the LES. Increased abdominal pressure may occur with obesity ("apple fat"), pregnancy, delayed gastric emptying or gastroparesis, overeating, constipation with build-up of stool in the large intestine, and sudden blows to the abdomen.

Trauma

Years ago, a patient told me that all his chronic digestive problems started after jumping off a high wall and landing hard on his feet. Another patient described how he had fallen from a tall tree, also landing feet first on the ground. The upward pressure from the hard landings caused hiatal hernia syndrome. Fortunately, I was able to correct both with a visceral massage technique discussed later in this chapter.

Breath Holding and Contracting Abdominal Muscles

Breath holding while contracting abdominal muscles is referred to as the Valsalva maneuver and is also relevant to hiatal hernias. Examples of breath holding include straining while bearing down during a bowel movement or while lifting a heavy object. Inhaling and then holding the breath during exertion/straining seems to create the highest pressures in the abdomen (Galmiche JP, 1995). Holding the breath during exertion feels natural because it can stabilize the spine and reduce the risk of herniated discs (Hagins M, 2006), but it also increases the risk of creating a variety of hernias. Both reduced LES tone and the presence of a hiatal hernia increase the likelihood of reflux episodes during the Valsalva maneuver (Sloan S et al, 1992). To reduce the risk of developing a hiatal hernia while exerting, see the "Treatment" section below.

Excess Gas

Another common cause of increased pressure leading to hiatal hernia is excess gas and distention in the small intestine. Contributing factors to excess gas are discussed in chapters nine (diets) and sixteen (SIBO).

Other Symptoms of Hiatal Hernia

Often, primary care physicians are unaware that symptoms other than reflux and regurgitation can be caused by hiatal hernias. There are, however, several symptoms that can indicate a hiatal hernia (Failor R, 1975 and Sandberg-Lewis S, 2017). These include:

- fatigue

- brain fog

- excessive fullness after consuming even small portions of food

- rapid shallow breathing

- a sensation of chest pressure or shortness of breath

- a feeling of fullness in the throat

- anxiety

- difficulty swallowing

- a chronic tickling cough

- an uncomfortable constricted sensation at the waist

HIATAL HERNIA SYNDROME VERSUS SLIDING HIATAL HERNIA

The term "hiatal hernia syndrome" is used when the symptoms of a sliding hiatal hernia are present and in-office tests indicate it is likely, but without confirmation by diagnostic imaging.

Examples of diagnostic imaging that can reveal a sliding hiatal hernia include an upper GI series (also called a barium swallow), an upper endoscopy, chest x-ray, or CT or MRI scans that involve both the abdomen and chest. Such imaging, along with tests of the heart and lungs, are sometimes important to rule out conditions that may have symptoms similar to hiatal hernia. Relatively simple reflex point or functional muscle tests can be used by health practitioners to check for hiatal hernia syndrome during an office visit. The good news is that many sliding hiatal hernias, as well as the syndrome itself, can be treated with manual techniques rather than surgery.

The uncommon paraesophageal hernia cannot be corrected as described below.

TREATMENTS

MANUAL MANIPULATIONS

There are various manual manipulation or massage techniques available to treat sliding hiatal hernia and hiatal hernia syndrome. Some require a more forceful downward thrust, known as the Failor technique, and others are gentler. I learned the thrust technique from Dr. Ralph Failor in the late 1970s, a method which is still used by many chiropractic physicians. In the mid-1990s, I studied other bodywork techniques such as structural integration and the Barral method. The skills I gained changed my approach to manipulation of the abdominal organs and I gradually developed the gentler techniques I now use. I teach them to other physicians and bodyworkers. For health care practitioners who wish to learn more, the hiatal hernia syndrome visceral manipulation technique is described in detail in chapter twelve of *Functional Gastroenterology: Assessing and Addressing the Causes of Functional Gastrointestinal Disorders*, 2nd edition.

Exercises You Can Do at Home

Heel Drops

Before eating in the morning, drink 12-16 ounces of water within 2 minutes, stand, rise onto the balls of your feet, and then drop onto the heels eleven (11) times in succession. The downward momentum of the water-filled pendulous stomach supports the benefits of previous visceral work. This practice is normally continued each morning for a minimum of fourteen days.

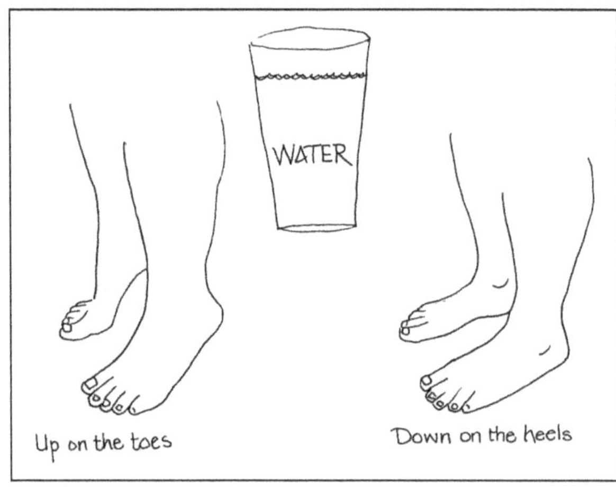

Fig. 12.4. Heel drop exercise.

Exercises for the Core

Core exercises are important to improve posture and abdominal muscle tone. One example that is safe for most beginners is the Knee Raise, illustrated here. While sitting in a chair, support the upper body by holding the arms or seat of the chair. Inhale, then exhale while pulling your legs toward your trunk as far as you can. Inhale again while extending your legs and rest your feet on the floor. Remember to exhale as you repeat the procedure.

Gradually increase repetitions over time.

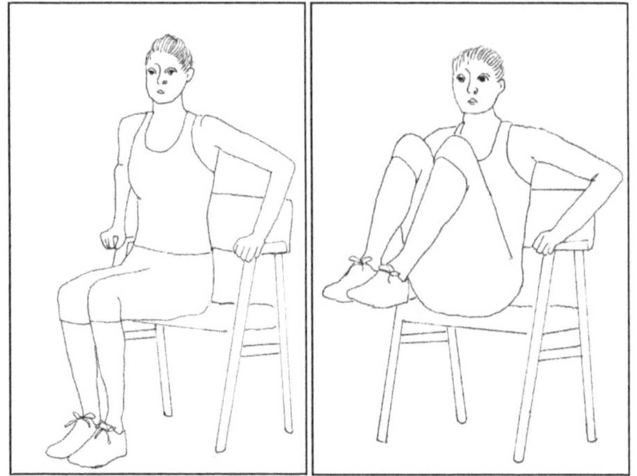

Fig. 12.5. Simple seated core exercise.

Dietary Basics

These vary with each person's individual needs. In general, I find that having my patients avoid their individual food sensitivities is important. Just as important as "what" they eat is "how" they eat.

- Avoid overeating and large meals
- Take time to sit and chew food until it becomes liquid before swallowing, (the term for this is Fletcherizing);
- Avoid stressful discussions or watching television while eating.

- If family of origin eating issues continue to affect your eating habits, consider counseling or energetic psychology interventions.

Treat hypochlorhydria or achlorhydria if present (see chapter fourteen).

BREATHING

Functional breathing is crucial. Learn to use functional diaphragmatic breathing when lifting, bearing down to have a bowel movement or during other exertion involving the abdominal muscles. Take a slow abdominal breath before exerting and then exhale as you lift or contract the abdominal muscles. This practice should be included when you are exercising, especially when doing crunches, sit ups and other core abdominal exercises. This technique will help prevent a build-up of intra-abdominal pressure, thus preventing reinjury. A video detailing diaphragmatic breathing can be found at www.hmmpdx.com/videos.

HIATAL HERNIA SYNDROME CASE EXAMPLE

Mary, a 47 year old woman, first came to my office with symptoms including heartburn, night time regurgitation, and a full sensation from her neck to the lower end of her sternum. She had an extensive history of vomiting that preceded the onset of frequent heartburn, brain fog and mild anxiety. She had not had an upper endoscopy or any GI workup. She had a long history of taking acid suppressive medicine. She reported that a proton pump inhibitor had relieved the throat symptoms, but had caused side effects and any benefits were short-lived.

I used my hiatal hernia syndrome visceral technique as well as some general freeing of the diaphragm and ribs by myofascial release. I instructed her to use the heel drop exercise each morning for at least two weeks following our visit. Checking in with her after I performed the hiatal hernia syndrome manipulation she reported "feeling great" with almost no heartburn symptoms, even after eating previously problematic foods. She found she no longer needed heartburn medicine.

Mary reported performing heel drops regularly. She confirmed coffee was a significant trigger for her heartburn. Dramatic improvement lasted for about three months. We had another visceral session at three months and then again after nine months. At the nine-month interval, Mary rated her recovery at 90%.

TREATMENT OF COMPLICATED CONDITONS

Unfortunately, due to lax soft tissue, people with hypermobility syndromes may have a more complex situation and visceral corrections may not stay in place for long. In other cases, complicated hiatal hernias may need surgical treatment for full resolution. These include larger hernias, wide openings in the diaphragm and the unusual form called paraesophageal hiatal hernia.

CITATIONS

Berkow R. Merck Manual, 18th ed, Merck and Co, April 2006

Smith AB, Dickerman RD, McGuire CS, East JW et al. Pressure-overload-induced sliding hiatal hernia in power athletes. J Clin Gastroenterol.1999 Jun;28(4):352-4. PMID: 10372935

Castori M, Morlino S, Pascolini G, Blundo C. Gastrointestinal and nutritional issues in joint hypermobility syndrome/ Ehlers-Danlos syndrome, hypermobility type. Am J Med Genet C Semin Med Genet. 2015 Mar;169C(1):54-75. PMID: 25821092

Menezes MA, Herbella FAM. Pathophysiology of Gastroesophageal Reflux Disease. World J Surg. 2017 Jul;41(7):1666-1671. PMID: 28258452. PMID: 28258452

Galmiche JP, Hanssens J. The pathophysiology of gastro-oesophageal reflux disease: an overview. Scand J Gastroenterol Suppl. 1995;211:7-18. PMID: 8545632

Hagins M, Lamberg EM. Natural breath control during lifting tasks: effect of load. Eur J Appl Physiol. 2006 Mar;96(4):453-8. PMID: 16341872

Sloan S, Rademaker AW, Kahrilas PJ. Determinants of gastroesophageal junction incompetence: hiatal hernia, lower esophageal sphincter, or both? Ann Intern Med. 1992 Dec 15;117(12):977-82. PMID: 1443984

Failor R, Three Generations of Healing Secrets ; Author, R. M. Failor ; Publisher, Failor, 1975 and The New Era Chiropractor, Self Published, 1979.

Sandberg-Lewis S, Functional Gastroenterology : Assessing and Addressing the Causes of Functional Digestive Disorders, Self-Published, 2017.

THIRTEEN

Helicobacter Pylori May Protect Against Reflux

H. pylori *is Jekyll or Hyde,*
Depends on the age you reside.
Preventing a zillion
Diseases in children,
Or later in life—health denied.

Glossary

antral gastritis—gastritis limited to the lower portion of the stomach

commensal—normal and often beneficial microorganisms in the body

gastritis—inflammation of the stomach lining

gastrobiome—beneficial organisms that live in the stomach

ghrelin—a hormone, produced mostly in the stomach, that increases appetite

lymphoma—cancer of the lymphatic system

MALToma—a form of lymphoma occurring in the stomach lining

pangastritis—gastritis affecting all three portions of the stomach

thrombocytopenia—low blood platelet count

KEY QUESTIONS

Is there anything good about *Helicobacter pylori*?

Is it true that *H. pylori* can be commensal?

Should I be tested for *H. pylori* because I have GERD?

Helicobacter pylori (*H. pylori*) is a spiral-shaped bacteria that lives in the human stomach. Every mammal on earth has a type of *Helicobacter* in its stomach. Pigs have *Helicobacter suis*, dolphins have *Helicobacter cetorum* and cheetahs have the difficult to pronounce *Helicobacter acinonyx*.

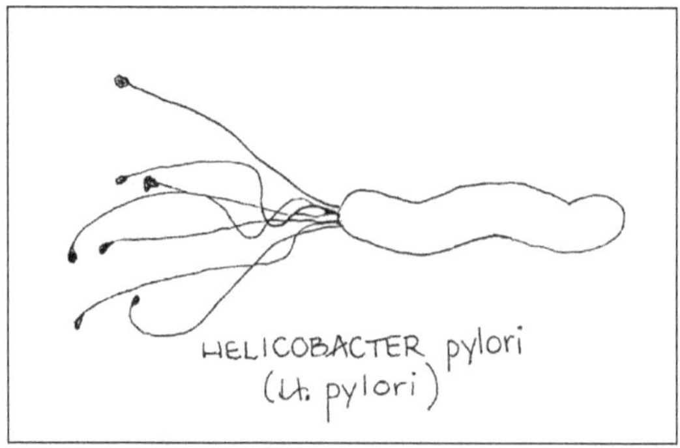

Fig. 13.1. *Helicobacter pylori*.

The human version of *Helicobacter*, *H. pylori*, has been with us for at least 58,000 years, and has migrated with its human host throughout the world. It is believed that prior to the era of antibiotics, virtually all of us had this bug as the predominant organism in our upper digestive system. If you are interested in reading more about the evolution of *Helicobacter* in humans, I recommend Martin Blaser's book entitled *Missing Microbes*. Dr. Blaser is a researcher and chair of microbiome studies at New York University and refers to *H. pylori* as an "ancient dominion organism".

In young children, H. pylori reduces the risk of developing the following diseases later in life: GERD, Barrett's esophagus, esophageal adenocarcinoma, asthma, hay fever, eczema, Crohn's disease, tuberculosis and cancer of the larynx.

Babies aren't born with this important organism. Instead, they rely on parents and siblings to introduce it to their **gastrobiome**. *H. pylori* may also be transmitted through water, soil, and saliva. In the newborn and young child, *H. pylori* reduces the risk of developing several infectious, allergic, and autoimmune diseases as well as cancers. Among these are asthma, hay fever, eczema, Crohn's disease, tuberculosis, and cancer of the larynx.

On the other hand, certain subtypes of *H. pylor*i are associated with **gastritis**, as well as peptic ulcers, stomach cancer and a rare form of **lymphoma** called **MALToma** which forms in the stomach. Because of those risks, this bacterial species has earned a "test and treat" approach in medicine, meaning whenever it is found on a test, it gets treated with various combinations of antibiotics and PPIs.

I don't advocate testing for *H. pylori* as a general screening for digestive issues. Current testing doesn't differentiate between **commensal** *H. pylori* and the type of *H. pylori* that can cause disease. The health benefits are not clear for testing and treating those with *H. pylori* who have reflux as their sole digestive diagnosis. Research suggests a connection between *H. pylori* treatment and an increase in reflux. This is especially an issue for people of Asian heritage (Xie T et al, 2013).

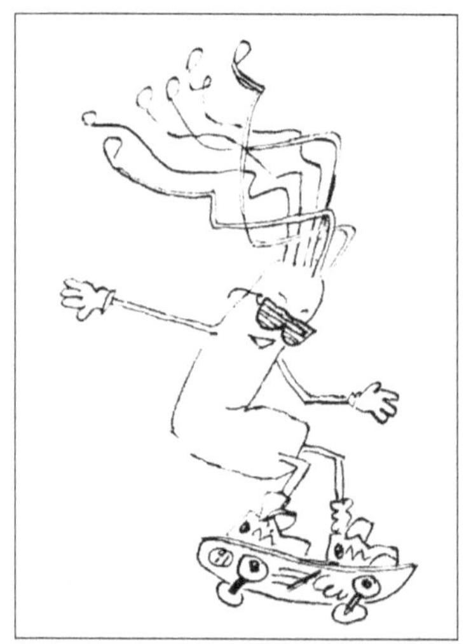

Fig. 13.2. Certain subtypes of *H. pylori* are associated with gastritis.

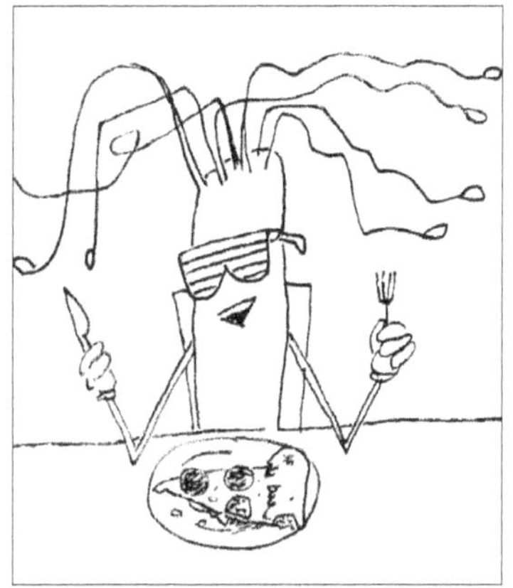

Fig. 13.3. *H. pylori* may be protective against reflux and its complications..

Our youngest citizens are the fifth generation to be frequently exposed to prescription antibiotics.

H. pylori may be protective against reflux and its complications, which include Barrett's esophagus, Barrett's with dysplasia, and esophageal cancer (Thrift AP, 2012; Mungan Z et al, 2017; Cook MB, 2021). Reflux may increase or decrease following *H. pylori* treatment (Yucel O, 2019). In addition, several patients have told me their symptoms of irritable bowel syndrome and small intestine bacterial overgrowth (SIBO) were triggered when they were treated for *H. pylori*.

Although the type of cancer associated with GERD, known as esophageal adenocarcinoma (EAC), was previously uncommon, over the second half of the 20th century, EAC became the most rapidly increasing cancer in the Western world. EAC occurs in areas affected by Barrett's esophagus. Barrett's develops in some people with a long history of GERD. Compared to the general population, having Barrett's is associated with a significant increase in risk for developing esophageal cancer. The good news is that EAC is not rising as rapidly as previously, and the odds are low that it will develop—only about 4 in100,000 people, and even rarer if you consider only women (Pohl H, 2010). Other risk factors for Barrett's and EAC include abdominal obesity, high dietary fat, and smoking (Snider EJ et al, 2016). More details on Barrett's are in chapter eighteen.

We are in the fifth generation of Americans commonly exposed to prescription antibiotic treatment. Research has suggested that repeated use of antibiotics to treat ear infections, bronchitis, etc, can eradicate *H. pylori* (Blaser MJ, 2011). The average child in the US has received 17 courses of antibiotics by age 20 (Blaser, MJ 2014).

The widespread and excessive use of antibiotics began in the 1940s and caused major shifts in the upper gastrointestinal microflora. The percentage of people with *H. pylori* in their stomachs began to decrease in the mid-20th century, corresponding with a soon-to-follow rise in EAC.

To understand the various effects of *H. pylori*, one must understand that location makes all the difference. It can behave as nature's proton pump inhibitor or stimulator depending on where it colonizes in the stomach. The condition called **pangastritis,** when *H. pylori* colonizes the entire stomach, tends to reduce gastric acid production, leading to reduced acid reflux. Interestingly, when it resides in only the lower portion of the stomach, causing **antral gastritis**, it tends to increase gastric acid and the risk of peptic ulcers. To clarify where in the stomach *H. pylori* has colonized, whether it is pangastritis or antral gastritis, an upper endoscopy must be performed. Standard tests, however, test for *H. pylori* using blood, breath, or stool samples. These tests cannot identify where in the stomach the *H. pylori* is colonized or whether there is gastritis. Upper endoscopy is a thorough and accurate way to make the necessary diagnosis.

Because less than 10% of the adult population in the US carry *H. pylori*, few parents can pass it on to their offspring (Sonnenberg A. et al 2020). People who have no *H. pylori* have higher levels of **ghrelin**, a hormone created in the stomach. Ghrelin increases appetite which can lead to obesity. Obesity is a risk factor for reflux (Bahar A, 2021).

Based on what I've written, the reader might assume that I believe *H. pylori* is always a normal part of the stomach's microbes and should never be treated. That is not my position. There are many good reasons for treating *H. pylori*, the best being peptic ulcers, especially if they are recurrent. MALToma has up to a 90% cure rate with full *H. pylori* treatment (Nakamura S 2013). Gastric cancer is a risk in about 1% of those with *H. pylori* pangastritis. Also, chronic iron deficiency and **thrombocytopenia** may be related to *H. pylori*, and therapy may normalize iron and platelet levels in such cases. On the other hand, evidence suggests protection from reflux in those who do have *H. pylori* in the stomach.

CITATIONS

Thrift AP et al, *Helicobacter pylori* infection and the risks of Barrett's esophagus: a population-based case-control study. Int J Cancer 2012 May 15;130(10):2407-16. PMID: 21681741.

Mungan Z, Pinarbasi Simsek BP. Gastroesophageal reflux disease and the relationship with Helicobacter pylori. Turk J Gastroenterol 2017; 28(Suppl 1): S61-S67. PMID: 29199171.

Xie T, Zheng H, Jiang B. Eradication of *H. pylori* may cause gastroesophageal reflux disease: a meta-analysis. Nan Fang Yi Ke Da Xue Xue Bao. 2013 May;33(5):719-23. PMID: 23688993.

Yucel O. Interactions between *Helicobacter pylori* and gastroesophageal reflux disease. Esophagus. 2019 Jan;16(1):52-62. PMID 30151653

Cook MB, Thrift AP. Epidemiology of Barrett's Esophagus and Esophageal Adenocarcinoma: Implications for Screening and Surveillance. Gastrointest Endosc Clin N Am. 2021 Jan;31(1):1-26. PMID: 33213789

Pohl H, Sirovich B, Welch HG. Esophageal adenocarcinoma incidence: are we reaching the peak? Cancer Epidemiol Biomarkers Prev. 2010;19(6):1468–70. PMID: 20501776.

Snider EJ, Freedberg DE, Abrams JA, Potential Role of the Microbiome in Barrett's Esophagus and Esophageal Adenocarcinoma. Dig Dis Sci. 2016 Aug; 61(8): 2217–2225. PMID: 27068172

Blaser M. Antibiotic overuse: Stop the killing of beneficial bacteria. Nature . 2011 Aug 24;476(7361):393-4. PMID: 21866137

Blaser MJ. Missing Microbes: How the Overuse of Antitbiotics Is Fueling Our Modern Plagues. Henry Holt and Company, 2014

Sonnenberg A, Turner KO, Genta RM. Low Prevalence of *Helicobacter pylori*-Positive Peptic Ulcers in Private Outpatient Endoscopy Centers in the United States. Am J Gastroenterol. 2020 Feb;115(2):244-250. PMID: 31972622

Bahar A, Mirmohammad Khani M, Dabiri R, Semnani V. *H. pylori* effects on ghrelin axis: Preliminary change in gastric pathogenesis. Microb Pathog. 2021 Dec;161(Pt A):105262. PMID: 34695557

Nakamura S, Matsumoto T. *Helicobacter pylori* and gastric mucosa-associated lymphoid tissue lymphoma: recent progress in pathogenesis and management. World J Gastroenterol. 2013 Dec 7;19(45):8181-7. PMID: 24363507

Epplein M, Signorella LB, Zheng W, Peek RM et al. Race, African ancestry, and Helicobacter pylori infection in a low-income United States population. Cancer Epidemiol Biomarkers Prev. 2011 May;20(5):826-34. PMID: 21357376

FOURTEEN

Too Much or Too Little Acid?

pH can vary a lot.
Get tested to see what you've got.
Assuming GERD's acid,
Is often deemed tacit,
But more often not what you thought.

Glossary

achlorhydria—the absence of acid in the stomach

applied kinesiology—a system used to evaluate health in part by correlating muscle strength with organ function

bicarbonate—a base (opposite of an acid) which prevents the body from becoming too acidic

cholecystitis—inflammation of the gall bladder lining

euchlorhydria—normal acid concentration in the stomach

Hashimoto's thyroiditis—an autoimmune disease in which the immune system attacks the thyroid gland, often leading to an underactive thyroid

hyperchlorhydria— increased level of stomach acid

hypochlorhydria—reduced level of stomach acid

myasthenia gravis—a rare chronic autoimmune disease marked by muscular weakness

rosacea—a condition in which certain facial blood capillaries enlarge, giving the cheeks nose or forehead a flushed appearance. Pimples may also form in these areas.

Sjogren's syndrome—a chronic autoimmune condition characterized by degeneration of the salivary and lachrymal glands, causing dryness of the mouth and eyes

vitiligo—a condition in which the pigment is lost from areas of the skin, causing pale patches

KEY QUESTIONS

What are the functions of gastric acid?

Is all heartburn due to excessive acid production?

How is stomach pH measured?

GASTRIC ACID

Gastric acid is crucial in the digestion of protein, folic acid, vitamin B12 and minerals. As the stomach empties its acid into the small intestine, the release of pancreatic enzymes and **bicarbonate** are stimulated. Gastric acid also helps reduce the level of bacteria, yeast and some parasites that enter the body through the mouth and, importantly, prevents the overgrowth of bacteria which can otherwise lead to small intestine bacterial overgrowth.

Hydrochloric acid is very potent. If you were to spill concentrated hydrochloric acid on your skin, it would burn the skin away. The membranes lining the esophagus, stomach and duodenum contain mucus cells and bicarbonate producing cells to protect themselves and neutralize some of the acid. Bicarbonate is an alkaline substance which reduces acidity—raising the acid pH closer to neutral. Neutral substances are the least irritating to the lining of the digestive tract because they are a similar pH to blood.

ACID LEVELS

Although it seems counterintuitive, the reduced levels of acid in **hypochlorhydria** often cause heartburn. Instead of producing excess stomach acid, most patients with heartburn produce either normal amounts of acid or too little. Over the last 25 years of Heidelberg testing, I have found that about half of heartburn sufferers have hypochlorhydria. **Hyperchlorhydria**—excessive stomach acid— has been found in only about a fifth of those I have tested.

Symptoms and Diseases Associated with Hypochlorhydria

Common symptoms of hypochlorhydria include heartburn; excessive gas, bloating, or burping; nausea; a sensation of fullness after consuming even small amounts of food, and/or a heavy sensation in the stomach after meals—as if food is sitting there and will not digest. This is especially true for meals containing concentrated protein. These same symptoms are also common signs of delayed gastric emptying because adequate acid is part of a group of factors that control the opening of the pyloric valve, allowing the stomach to gradually empty.

Diseases associated with deficient gastric acid levels include: diabetes, iron and B12 deficiency anemia, rheumatoid arthritis, autoimmune hepatitis, **myasthenia gravis**, **Sjogren's syndrome**, hypothyroidism, and **Hashimoto's thyroiditis**. Additionally, other diseases, such as stomach inflammation (chronic atrophic gastri-tis), and some skin diseases, such as psoriasis, **alopecia**, chronic hives, eczema, **vitiligo**, and **rosacea**, often occur along with hypo-chlorhydria (Rodriguez-Castro KI, 2018).

MEASURING STOMACH ACID LEVELS

HEIDELBERG TEST

Reflux of stomach contents into the lower esophagus is best mea-sured with pH impedance testing, but the direct pH of the stom-ach itself is measured using the Heidelberg machine. The Hei-delberg test involves swallowing a small capsule as described in chapter four.

GENERAL INDICATORS OF GASTRIC ACID LEVELS

Functional markers for hypochlorhydria or hyperchlorhydria

Your healthcare practitioner may note functional markers that suggest the presence of hypochlorhydria. These physical exam markers may point to the need for further testing. I find these tests helpful to check body circuits related to stomach pH. They are _not_ diagnostic. They are generally employed by certain natu-ropathic, osteopathic, and chiropractic physicians as well as some acupuncturists.

Additional physical signs may be present.

- a tendency to have soft, brittle, or peeling nails

- generalized thinning of scalp hair in women

- dilated, tortuous blood vessels over the cheekbones, chin, or mid forehead, although this may also be a sign of rosacea, which can be associated with other diges-tive problems such as small intestine bacterial over-growth (SIBO) and Crohn's disease

- a heavily coated tongue and/or bad breath

Riddler's gastric acid point

Robert Riddler, DC, ND identified a reflex point located on the low-er left margin of the ribcage, which if tender can indicate that lev-els of gastric acid are either excessive or deficient. The presence of tenderness does not, however, differentiate between the two states of acidity. Instead, it can be a quick way to test a hypothesis.

Applied kinesiology

George Goodheart, DC is attributed with the **applied kinesiology** testing of the pectoralis major clavicular muscles (PMC). When neither the right nor left PMC "lock" properly on strength testing, hypochlorhydria may be investigated further. This is one of many kinesiology tests for the stomach and is considered a general indicator of a decreased production of stomach acid.

Other functional tests include acid trials

The vinegar challenge

The simplest test you can try is a vinegar challenge. If eating foods containing vinegar does not aggravate your heartburn, you may try the following.

- Mix 1-2 teaspoonfuls of apple cider vinegar in a ¼ cup of water.

- Drink 10-15 minutes prior to a meal.

Many people with hypochlorhydria find this helps their digestion and reduces heartburn symptoms. If it makes your symptoms worse, do not repeat. If it is helpful, it could be a way for you to improve your stomach acid production. If taken before each meal and if done long term, however, please take care of your dental enamel by using a straw so the vinegar does not directly bathe the teeth. Another option is to brush or thoroughly rinse the teeth with water after swallowing the vinegar solution.

Medicinal bitter herbs

Another trial uses medicinal bitter herbs (as opposed to bitters used in creating cocktails) to assist normal acid production. Bitter herbs have many functions besides acid production and may prove helpful for other aspects of digestion.

Typical use of tincture of bitter herbs includes

- Four drops of bitters tincture on the tongue before meals or

- 10 -15 drops of bitters in a quarter cup of water, swallowed before meals

Betaine hydrochloride capsules

Yet another acid trial uses betaine hydrochloride capsules, typically with added pepsin. Some physicians and nutritionists use a trial of these capsules to provide a certain amount of hydrochloric acid during meals as a practical way to see if hypochlorhydria is present. If you know that you have active gastritis, peptic ulcer or erosive esophagitis, this trial is not recommended. In my practice, I use the Heidelberg test to determine whether hypochlorhydria is present. Betaine hydrochloride or bitter herbs may be swallowed during the Heidelberg test if hypochlorhydria is found. This allows a direct reading of the effect of bitters or betaine hydrochloride on the gastric pH of the patient being tested.

CITATIONS

Rodriguez-Castro Kryssia I, Marilisa F, Antonino N, Chiara M et al. Clinical manifestations of chronic atrophic gastritis. Acta Biomed,2018; 89(Suppl 8): 88–92. PMID: 30561424

FIFTEEN

PANCREATIC INSUFFICIENCY AND GERD

When the pancreas fails to produce
Enough of the right kinds of juice,
It's hard to break down
Chyme in Duoden Town.
Malabsorption may make the stools loose.

GLOSSARY

amino acids—the chemical building blocks of proteins

amylase—a pancreatic enzyme that digests starches into sugars

bile stasis (also called cholestasis)—a decrease in the flow of bile through the liver or bile ducts

brush border enzymes—enzymes produced by the lining of the small intestine that complete the last step in digestion of carbohydrates and proteins

chymotrypsin—a pancreatic enzyme that digests protein

cow's milk protein enteropathy—a cause of persistent diarrhea and malabsorption in young infants fed cow's milk formula

elastase—a pancreatic enzyme that digests protein

endocrine—glands that secrete hormones or other substances directly into the blood

exocrine—glands that secrete their products through ducts opening onto the lining membrane of an organ

exocrine pancreatic insufficiency (EPI)—a condition in which there are not enough pancreatic digestive enzymes to properly digest fat, protein and carbohydrate foods

glutathione peroxidase—an enzyme that protects cells from oxidative damage

hemochromatosis—a hereditary disorder in which iron is deposited in the tissues, which if not treated early, can cause type I diabetes, damage to the liver and pancreas, and other diseases

lipase—a pancreatic enzyme that digests fat

pancreatic acini—structures in the pancreas that produce, store and release digestive enzymes

peptides—short fragments of protein, two or three amino acids long

porcine—referring to pigs

proteases—enzymes that digest protein

secretin—a hormone produced in the duodenum that stimulates the pancreas to release enzymes and bicarbonate.

short bowel syndrome—the loss of greater than 50% of functioning small intestine due to disease or surgery

trypsin—a pancreatic enzyme that digests protein

KEY QUESTIONS

What are the functions of pancreatic digestive enzymes and bicarbonate?

How does reduced production of pancreatic digestive enzymes affect reflux?

What digestive problems are associated with EPI?

Pancreatic Functions

Tucked beneath the stomach, the pancreas is a digestive organ that is often misunderstood. Most patients associate the pancreas with insulin and diabetes, but it has many more functions. It is comprised of two parts: The digestive, or **exocrine** portion produces enzymes and bicarbonate while the hormonal or **endocrine** portion produces insulin and other hormones. For our purposes, we will focus on its exocrine aspects. The pancreas is unique among gastrointestinal organs because it produces enzymes that are involved in digesting all three major nutrients—fats, proteins, and carbohydrates. The enzymes are made in **pancreatic acini**, drain into the pancreatic duct, and eventually empty into the small intestine.

To review, the digestive route prior to the intestine:

After food is chewed and swallowed, the bolus travels down the esophagus and enters the stomach within seconds. In the stomach, where the bolus becomes chyme, proteins in the food are broken down by acid and pepsin. This results in **peptides** which are short chains of **amino acids**. There is no digestion of carbohydrates and only minimal digestion of fats in the stomach. Over a four-to-five-hour period, the chyme gradually leaves the stomach and enters the first part of the small intestine, the duodenum.

Regulating pH

There is a lot going on in the duodenum and much of it is due to the secretions of the pancreas. First, the pH of the acidic chyme from the stomach must be neutralized. If not, too much acid will damage the duodenal lining and inactivate

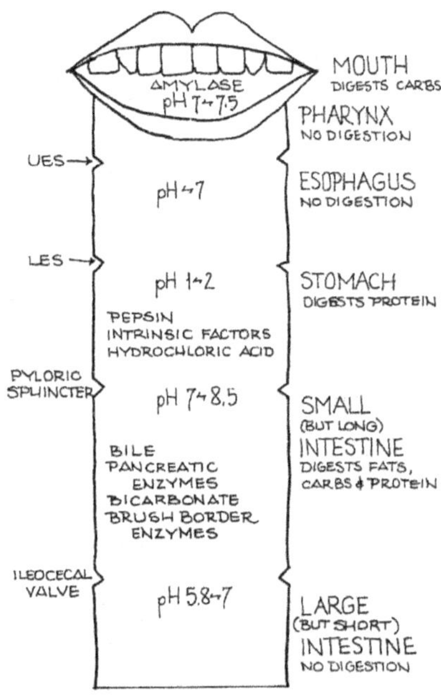

Fig 15.1. Pancreatic enzymes in the sequence of digestive secretions.

pancreatic enzymes. To prevent this from happening, the pancreas releases bicarbonate which quickly changes the pH from a strong acid to a very weak acid.

DIGESTIVE ENZYMES

The pancreas produces many enzymes. These include **trypsin**, **elastase**, and **chymotrypsin** for protein digestion, **amylase** for carbohydrate digestion, and **lipase** for fat digestion. Testing stool samples for levels of elastase (an alternative test is stool chymotrypsin) is how we determine pancreatic digestive function. When stool elastase levels are below 200 ug/mL, a diagnosis of pancreatic exocrine insufficiency (EPI)* is made (Kampanis P, 2009). Exocrine pancreatic insufficiency occurs when the exocrine portion of the pancreas is unable to create enough enzymes to properly digest food.

CAUSES AND EFFECTS OF EXOCRINE PANCREATIC INSUFFICIENCY

SIBO AND GAS PRODUCTION

As part of a series of balancing measures, pancreatic enzymes also control the growth of small intestinal bacteria and other microorganisms. The most likely relationship between pancreatic insufficiency and reflux is SIBO. One third of patients with chronic pancreatitis, which often causes EPI, test positive for SIBO using a glucose breath test (Capurso, 2016). In fact, a recent research paper found that fasting hydrogen levels were 5-fold higher in subjects with EPI compared to controls. Uetsuki K et al. have suggested using a single fasting hydrogen breath testing as a screening test for EPI (Uetsuki, 2021). High gas production in the small intestine increases intra-abdominal pressure which, in turn, may increase the risk of GERD.

BEHAVIORAL FACTORS

Behaviors associated with pancreatic insufficiency include tobacco use, excessive alcohol consumption and excessive consumption of simple carbohydrates.

---

*Note: Some researchers and journals use the abbreviation PEI, or pancreatic exocrine insufficiency.

DISEASES

Diseases that can be underlying causes of exocrine pancreatic insufficiency include

- chronic viral hepatitis
- short bowel syndrome
- hemochromatosis
- partial surgical removal of the stomach or pancreas
- pancreatic cancer
- celiac disease
- chronic pancreatitis
- bile stasis
- cystic fibrosis
- casein (milk protein) and gluten intolerance
- hypochlorhydria
- types I and II diabetes mellitus

INSULIN LEVELS

EPI occurs in about 50% of insulin dependent diabetics and 30-50% of non-insulin dependent diabetics (Hardt DH, 2011 and Hardt PD, 2003). Diabetics also have a high rate of GERD (Sun XM, 2015). EPI is more common in people who are obese, have elevated blood fats or insulin resistance (Chonchubhair, 2018 and Vesterhus, 2008).

30–50% of diabetics have EPI. Diabetics also have a high rate of GERD.

HEPATITIS B AND C

Chronic viral hepatitis B or C can also cause pancreatic insufficiency, as shown by a Russian study that found enzyme deficiency in 18% of viral hepatitis patients (Wasielica-Berger, 2007 and Shamychkova AA, 2006).

Celiac Disease and EPI

It is estimated that more than 20% of patients with celiac disease have EPI (Leeds JS, 2007). Celiac disease is also more common in those with diabetes, which was discussed above as another risk factor for EPI (Freeman HJ, 2007). People who consume gluten despite active celiac disease will have a reduction of villi, the finger shaped protrusions lining the small intestine. Blunting or total loss of villi greatly reduces the surface area of the intestine

20% of patients with celiac disease also have EPI.

needed for nutrient absorption. When people with typical celiac disease consume gluten, partial or total villous atrophy occurs, leaving a nearly flat surface. This results in protein deficiency, leading to loss of pancreatic glands and deficient enzyme synthesis.

Children with both EPI and celiac disease no longer had EPI after eating a gluten-free diet for 12 months.

There is evidence, however, that patients who maintain a fully gluten free diet for at least 12 months have healed pancreatic insufficiency. A study of children with celiac disease found that enzyme production and the structure of the intestinal lining returned to normal after following a gluten-free diet for twelve months (Carroccio A,1991).

FACTORS TO CONSIDER FOR SUCCESSFUL EPI TREATMENT

Either an excessively acidic intestinal pH or bacterial overgrowth may prevent adequate fat digestion. These problems should be considered when a patient fails to respond to treatment for pancreatic insufficiency (Domínguez-Muñoz, 2007). The pH of the upper small intestine also controls the function of pancreatic enzymes, the ideal range being 6.8 to 8.0. Hyperchlorhydria or decreased bicarbonate production may increase the acidity of the duodenum which inactivates pancreatic enzymes. A pH below 4.5 will inactivate amylase, a pancreatic enzyme that digests starch into sugar, and lipase, a fat digestive enzyme.

Fat digestion in the small intestine starts with bile. Produced in the liver, bile is transported to the gall bladder where it is stored. When a fatty meal leaves the stomach, the gallbladder contracts and releases bile into the upper small intestine. The bile functions as an emulsifier the way soap acts on grease, breaking fat down to many small droplets. The small size of the droplets gives lipase the surface area it needs to digest the fat. Bacteria in the small intestine convert bile into a form that is less effective for emulsifying fat. In this way, bacterial overgrowth may cause fat malabsorption even when the pancreatic enzymes are not deficient.

TREATMENT OPTIONS IN PANCREATIC INSUFFICIENCY*

PANCREATIC ENZYME SUPPLEMENTS

Three main approaches are available.

Animal-based extracts

1. Pancreatin and pancrealipase contain a mix of amylase, lipase and proteases and are derived from **porcine** pancreas. These are taken after meals because their activity begins in the duodenum, and they work best at a near neutral pH. The prescription brand names Pancreaze and Viokase may be prescribed with PPIs to protect them from inactivation from gastric acidity.

Enterically coated animal-based extracts

2. These prescription formulations are enterically coated with phthalates to protect the pH sensitive enzymes from stomach acid. Brand names include Creon and Zenpep. These may be very effective especially for patients who have adequate acid production. Unfortunately, some phthalates have been proven to act as endocrine disruptors leading to altered thyroid and reproductive hormone levels (Gallinger ZR, 2013). Other medications containing phthalates include mesalamine, sulfasalazine, ranitidine, delayed release forms of omeprazole, bisacodyl (brand name Dulcolax) and some probiotic supplements used by gastroenterologists. More research is needed to study whether exposure to phthalates from medications will have negative consequences.

Plant-based enzymes

3. Plant based enzymes contain a mix of amylase, lipase and proteases and are derived from Aspergillus niger, a common fungus and therefore, are fungal enzymes. Active in a wide pH range from 2-12, this form of enzyme supplement is taken before meals because it is active in both the stomach and the duodenum. Various formulations may also contain additional **brush border enzymes** such as lactase, cellulase, sucrase, isomaltose and maltase.

   Papain, derived from papaya, and bromelain, derived from pineapple, are also excellent sources of plant **proteases**.

---

*A detailed presentation of diagnostic and treatment options for pancreatic insufficiency is given in my textbook, *Funtional Gastroenterology* (2017).

	TABLE 15.1. COMPARISON OF PORCINE AND PLANT (FUNGAL) ENZYMES			
ENZYME	SOURCE	OPTIMAL pH RANGE	DIGESTION BEGINS	WHEN TAKEN
Pancreatin or Pancrealipase	Porcine	6.8 – 8.0	In the duodenum	with or after meals
Plant based enzymes	Aspergillus niger	2.0-12.0	In the stomach	before meals

ORGANOTHERAPY

Homeopathically prepared pancreas referred to as pancreatinum, or homeopathic medicine derived from vagus nerve referred to as nervinum vagum, are used by some health practitioners to stimulate exocrine pancreatic function.

ANTIOXIDANT NUTRITION

Antioxidants are found at lower levels in patients with pancreatic insufficiency than in the general population. Patients with moderate to severe chronic pancreatitis were found to have significantly lower mean selenium levels than controls (Vaona, 2005). Those with alcoholism induced chronic pancreatitis had significantly reduced blood levels of vitamin E, vitamin A, selenium, and **glutathione peroxidase** compared to controls with similar dietary intakes of these essential antioxidant nutrients (Van Gossum A, 1996).

CITATIONS

Capurso G et al. Systematic review and meta-analysis: Small intestinal bacterial overgrowth in chronic pancreatitis. United European Gastroenterol J. 2016 Oct;4(5):697-705. PMID: 27733912

Uetsuki, K et al. Measurement of fasting breath hydrogen concentration as a simple diagnostic method for pancreatic exocrine insufficiency. BMC Gastroenterol. 2021 May 10;21(1):211. PMID: 33971823

Hardt, DH, Nils E. Exocrine pancreatic insufficiency in diabetes mellitus: a complication of diabetic neuropathy or different type of diabetes? Exp Diabetes Res 2011; 2011; 761950. PMID: 21822421

Sun XM, Tan JC, Zhu Y, Lin L. Association between diabetes mellitus and gastroesophageal reflux disease: a meta-analysis. World J Gastroenterol 2015; 21: 3085-92. PMID: 25780309

Chonchubhair HMN et al. The prevalence of small intestinal bacterial overgrowth in non-surgical patients with chronic pancreatitis and pancreatic exocrine insufficiency (PEI), Pancreatology. 2018 Jun;18(4):379-385. PMID: 29502987

Vesterhus, M et al. Pancreatic exocrine dysfunction in maturity-onset diabetes of the young type 3. Diabetes Care. 2008 Feb;31(2):306-10. PMID: 17989309

Hardt, PD et al. High prevalence of exocrine pancreatic insufficiency in diabetes mellitus. A multicenter study screening fecal elastase 1 concentrations in 1,021 diabetic patients. Dig Dis Sci. 2003 Sep;48(9):1688-92. PMID: 14526149

Wasielica-Berger J, Długosz JW, Łaszewicz W, Baniukiewicz A et al. Exocrine pancreatic function in biliary tract pathology treated with the endoscopic methods. Adv Med Sci. 2007;52:222-7. PMID: 18217422

Shamychkova AA, Nikushkin EV. The activity of gastrointestinal enzymes in chronic viral hepatitis B and C] Klin Lab Diagn. 2006 Mar;(3):16-8. PMID: 16749485

Carroccio A, Iacono G, Montalto G, Cavataio F, Di Marco C, Balsamo V, Notarbartolo A. Exocrine pancreatic function in children with celiac disease before and after a gluten free diet. Gut. 1991 Jul;32(7):796-9. PMID:1855688.

Leeds JS, Hopper AD, Hurlstone DP, Edwards SJ et al. Is exocrine pancreatic insufficiency in adult coeliac disease a cause of persisting symptoms? Aliment Pharmacol Ther. 2007 Feb 1;25(3):265-71. PMID: 17269988

Freeman HJ. Pancreatic endocrine and exocrine changes in celiac disease. World J Gastroenterol. 2007 Dec 21;13(47):6344-6. PMID: 18081222

Nousia-Arvanitakis S, Fotoulaki M, Tendzidou K, Vassilaki C et al. Subclinical exocrine pancreatic dysfunction resulting from decreased cholecystokinin secretion in the presence of intestinal villous atrophy. J Pediatr Gastroenterol Nutr. 2006 Sep;43(3):307-12. PMID: 16954951

Hilgendorf I, Gellersen O, Emmrich J, Mikkat U et al. Estradiol has a direct impact on the exocrine pancreas as demonstrated by enzyme and vigilin expression. Pancreatology. 2001;1(1):24-9. PMID: 12120263

Morales-Miranda A, Robles-Díaz G, Díaz-Sánchez V. Steroid hormones and pancreas: a new paradigm] Rev Invest Clin. 2007 Mar-Apr;59(2):124-9. PMID: 17633800

Sandberg-Lewis S, Assessing and Addressing the Causes of Functional Gastrointestinal Disease, 2017 Mar, self-published.

Gallinger ZR, Nguyen GC, Presence of phthalates in gastrointestinal medications: is there a hidden danger? World J Gastroenterol. 2013 Nov 7;19(41):7042-7. PMID: 24222946

Domínguez-Muñoz JE Pancreatic enzyme therapy for pancreatic exocrine insufficiency. Curr Gastroenterol Rep. 2007 Apr;9(2):116-22. PMID: 17218056

Kampanis P, Ford L, Berg J. Development and validation of an improved test for the measurement of human faecal elastase-1. Ann Clin Biochem. 2009 Jan;46(Pt 1):33-7. PMID: 19008259

Vaona B, Stanzial AM, Talamini G, Bovo P et al. Serum selenium concentrations in chronic pancreatitis and controls. Dig Liver Dis. 2005 Jul;37(7):522-5. PMID: 15975540

Van Gossum A, Closset P, Noel E, Cremer M, Neve J. Deficiency in antioxidant factors in patients with alcohol-related chronic pancreatitis. Dig Dis Sci. 1996 Jun;41(6):1225-31. PMID: 8654156

SIXTEEN

SMALL INTESTINE BACTERIAL OVERGROWTH, GERD, AND THE PRESSURE DIFFERENTIAL

Bloating never feels very good
Because flora is eating your food.
They make many gases,
And until it all passes,
You'll be in a very bad mood.

GLOSSARY

adhesions—bands of scar tissue between two serosal surfaces (such as the outer layer of the intestines) that are not normally connected

anaerobes—organisms that grow without air or require oxygen-free conditions to live

archaea—single celled microorganisms, some of which can produce methane in the gut

autonomic neuropathy—damage to the nerves that control automatic body functions such as gut motility

biliary dyskinesia—a condition in which there is abnormal contractile activity of the gallbladder

blind loop—areas of intestine that lead to a dead end rather than continued movement of food and waste

body mass index—a measure of body fat based on height and weight

cecoileal—referring to the first portion of the large intestine and the last portion of the small intestine

colonic redundancy—the presence of an unusually lengthy large intestine

commensal—an organism living in and using food supplied by its host without damaging the host

Crohn's disease—a chronic inflammatory condition of the digestive tract, most commonly involving the small intestine

deep vein thrombosis—the formation of clots in the more internal veins of the leg

diverticulitis—inflammation of diverticular pouches that may form in the gut

duodenal duplication—when a child is born with more than one duodenum

endometriosis—a condition in which uterine lining tissue is found outside the uterus

failure to thrive—arrested physical growth (height and weight measurements) in children

fermentation—the transformation of carbohydrates into gas and heat by bacteria or yeast

ferritin—a protein that stores iron in body tissues

flocculation—the formation of small clumps of barium during an upper GI barium x-ray test

flora—plant, bacterial, or fungal organisms

gastroparesis—also called delayed gastric emptying, is a disorder that slows the movement of food from the stomach to the small intestine, even though there is no blockage in the stomach or intestines

glucose—a simple sugar which is a component of many carbohydrates

hepatic encephalopathy—a nervous system disorder brought on by severe liver disease. When the liver can't clear waste products properly,` excess ammonia can affect brain function.

interstitial cystitis—inflammation in the structure of the bladder causing pelvic pain or pressure and the frequent urge to urinate

intestinal methanogen overgrowth (IMO)—excessive numbers of organisms in the intestinal tract that convert hydrogen gas to methane gas

intracranial pressure—the pressure within the skull

irritable bowel syndrome—a functional disorder of the intestines marked by abdominal pain, bloating, and changes in bowel habits

lactulose—an indigestible sugar used as a laxative or as a test substance in SIBO breath testing

laparoscopic—a form of surgery performed in the abdomen or pelvis employing small incisions to insert a camera and surgical devices.

metabolic products—compounds produced by cells and excreted to the outside of the cell

metabolic syndrome—a cluster of risk factors that increase the risk of diabetes, heart disease and stroke. These include increased abdominal girth, high blood pressure, triglycerides, glucose and insulin as well as decreased high density lipoprotein (HDL)

microscopic colitis—a form of large intestine inflammation that causes copious non-bloody diarrhea. Not visible on the visual portion of a colonoscopy exam, it is diagnosed by colonic biopsy.

Nissen fundoplication— a surgery for the correction of reflux caused by sliding hiatal hernia

non-alcoholic steatohepatitis—inflammation of the liver due to excess fat deposition in the liver cells. It is associated with insulin resistance and diabetes.

pancreatitis—inflammation of the pancreas

prebiotics—various carbohydrates that are food sources for intestinal bacteria

prolapse—a downward displacement of a part or organ of the body from its normal position

proximal—located closer to the beginning rather than the end of the digestive tract

rosacea—dilated vessels and inflammation of the skin on the cheeks, chin or forehead.

scleroderma—an autoimmune disease marked by thickening of collagen in skin and the digestive tract

small bowel follow-through imaging—a series of x-rays using barium to provide contrast images for examination of the small intestine

small intestine bacterial overgrowth—excessive numbers of bacteria in the small intestine that produce hydrogen or hydrogen sulfide gas

small intestine diverticula—abnormal outpouchings in the small bowel

strictures—scar-like bands that develop on the inner lining of digestive organs, narrowing the opening

KEY QUESTIONS

What is SIBO?

How common is SIBO in GERD that is resistant to standard treatment?

How is increased intra-abdominal pressure related to SIBO and GERD?

39% of patients who did not respond to standard GERD treatment were found to have SIBO. 35% had IMO.

The use of proton pump inhibitors can cause SIBO and IMO.

People with a diagnosis of irritable bowel syndrome (IBS) often are not relieved of their symptoms after treatment. Their bloating, abdominal pain, constipation and/or diarrhea may continue. I have found that many of these patients have overgrowth of the normal beneficial **flora** in the small intestine. This chapter details the complex issues of small intestine bacterial overgrowth (SIBO) and intestinal methanogen overgrowth (IMO) and their relationships to GERD.

SIBO and IMO, previously called hydrogen dominant SIBO and methane dominant SIBO, are conditions in which the normally occurring beneficial bacteria or **archaea** grow beyond their normal numbers. SIBO/IMO is a common cause of **irritable bowel syndrome (IBS)**—in fact it is involved in over half the cases of IBS (Peralta S, 2009) and as high as 84% in one study using breath testing as the diagnostic marker (Lin HC, 2004.) It accounts for 37% of cases when cultures of fluid from the small intestine are used for diagnosis (Pyleris E, 2012.) Eradication of this overgrowth leads to a 75% reduction in IBS symptoms (Pimentel M, 2003).

WHY SIBO AND IMO MATTER IN REFLUX

In the context of our focus on reflux, considering a patient's SIBO/IMO diagnosis is important because having these gases can cause GERD that is resistant to treatment. In a recent study of patients with treatment resistant GERD, 39.4% had SIBO and 35.6% had IMO (Haworth JJ, 2021). These patients had been referred to surgeons specializing in **Nissen fundoplication**, a **laparoscopic surgery** used for treatment resistant reflux**.** Most fundoplication candidates have taken proton pump inhibitors (PPIs) for an average of over eight years. PPI use is one of the causes of SIBO/ IMO (Jacobs C, 2013). Research suggests that PPIs have a more profound altering effect on intestinal microbiota than antibiotics or any other class of drug (Imhann F, 2016). PPIs may allow the normal bacterial flora found in the mouth to travel down the gut and become dominant in the small intestine. While GI surgeons perform extensive testing to confirm reflux is the correct diagnosis before performing fundoplication surgery, testing for SIBO/IMO is not a part of their workups.

Bacterial or archaeal overgrowth leads to impairment of digestion and absorption and produces excess quantities of hydrogen, hydrogen sulfide and/or methane gas. Hydrogen and methane are not produced by human cells but are the **metabolic products** of intestinal organisms fermenting carbohydrates. When **commensals** (oral, small intestine or large intestine flora) multiply in the small intestine to excessive numbers, IBS, and subsequently reflux, become more likely.

Hydrogen/methane breath testing is the most widely used diagnostic method for this condition. Breath testing for both gases in SIBO (hydrogen and hydrogen sulfide) as well as methane gas in IMO are also available. Typically, these tests use either **glucose** or **lactulose** solutions to provide sugar for the microorganisms to ferment into gas. Some research directly cultures bacteria from the duodenum (collected during an upper endoscopy procedure) to diagnose SIBO/IMO. When reviewing the research results, it is essential to note the type of testing used to make the diagnosis. Duodenal/jejunal sampling and glucose breath testing measure **proximal** SIBO only. Lactulose breath testing measures bacterial/archaeal overgrowth anywhere in the bowel (Pimentel M, 2012) Stool analysis has no value in diagnosing SIBO.

Symptoms of SIBO include:
- bloating/ abdominal gas
- flatulence, belching
- abdominal pain, discomfort, or cramps
- constipation, diarrhea, or a mixture of the two
- heartburn
- nausea
- malabsorption of fat; iron, vitamin A, D, E or B12 deficiency with or without anemia; and osteoporosis (Anantharaju A, 2003).
- systemic symptoms—headache, fatigue, joint or muscle pain and certain skin conditions

A partial list of other diseases associated with SIBO/IMO includes:
- erosive esophagitis (Kim KM, 2012)

- hypothyroidism (Lauritano EC, 2007)
- lactose intolerance (Almeida JA, 2008)
- gallstones (Kaur J, 2014)
- **Crohn's disease** (Klaus J, 2009)
- **scleroderma** (Marie I, 2009)
- celiac disease (Rubio-Tapia A 2009)
- chronic pancreatitis (Mancilla AC, 2008)
- **diverticulitis** (Tursi A, 2005)
- diabetes with **autonomic neuropathy** (Ojetti V, 2009)
- fibromyalgia and chronic regional pain syndrome (Goebel A, 2008)
- **hepatic encephalopathy** (Gupta A, 2010)
- **non-alcoholic steatohepatitis** (Shanab AA, 2011)
- **interstitial cystitis** (Weinstock LB, 2007)
- restless leg syndrome (Weinstock LB, 2011)
- **rosacea** (Parodi A, 2008)
- **deep vein thrombosis** (Fialho A, 2016)
- Based on my clinical experience, I suspect that some cases of **biliary dyskinesia** and **microscopic colitis** may also be associated with SIBO/IMO.

As mentioned above, malabsorption is a major concern and many of my patients are underweight based on their **body mass index** (**BMI**) scores. In the developing world this may be a major factor in **failure to thrive** and increased pediatric mortality (Donowitz JR, 2015).

The following clues increase my suspicion that a patient has SIBO/IMO:

- When a patient develops IBS following a bout of food poisoning or traveler's diarrhea (post-infectious IBS)
- When a patient reports dramatic transient improvement in IBS symptoms after antibiotic treatment for an unrelated infection
- When a patient reports worsening of IBS symptoms from ingesting probiotic supplements which also contain ***prebiotics***. This increase in symptoms occurs because prebiotics are carbohydrates that feed microorganisms, allowing more production of gas.

- When a patient reports that eating more fiber increases constipation and other IBS symptoms. Fiber is also fermented by microorganisms into gas.

- When a celiac patient reports insufficient improvement in digestive symptoms even when carefully following a gluten-free diet

- When a patient develops constipation type IBS (IBS-C) after taking narcotics

- When a patient has a chronic low **ferritin** level with no other apparent cause. Microorganisms take up iron, preventing their host from absorbing it.

- When IBS occurs in women who suffer from **endometriosis**

- When abdominal diagnostic imaging reveals a large gas accumulation obscuring the pancreas

- When **small bowel follow-through imaging** reveals areas of "flocculation" (Pimentel M, 2014)

MECHANISMS PROMOTING OVERGROWTH

Surprisingly, one research study suggests that surgical removal of the gall bladder reduces the risk of SIBO (Gabbard SL, 2014), but my clinical experience is that most abdominal or pelvic surgeries, as well as endometriosis, increase the risk of intestinal **adhesions.** Adhesions generally interrupt the smooth functioning of the migrating motor complex (MMC). The MMC is the small intestinal cleansing wave which is important for preventing overgrowth.

The use of proton pump inhibitors encourages overgrowth, especially of hydrogen producing bacteria (Pyleris E, 2012 and Jacobs C, 2013). See Fig. 16.1. for a more extensive listing of SIBO and IMO causes.

COMMON ORGANISMS THAT OVERGROW

The most common bacteria to be found overgrown in the small intestine are *Escherichia coli*, *Enterococcus* and *Klebsiella* species (Takakura W, 2020). In the large intestine, hydrogen production is believed to have **antioxidant** effects (Carbonero F, 2012) whereas excessive small intestine hydrogen causes the symptoms and signs of diarrhea type irritable bowel syndrome (IBS-D.)

Methanobrevibacter smithii (*M. smithii*) is the organism that,

The most common types of bacteria that overgrow in the small intestine are E. coli, Enterococcus and Klebsiella species.

when overgrown, causes IMO. *M. smithii* is found in the digestive tracts of 30-62% of humans. It converts hydrogen to methane and has also been linked to obesity (Million M, 2013).

Sulphate reducing bacteria, such as *Desulfovibrio* species, are **anaerobes** that combine hydrogen with sulfur to produce hydrogen sulfide. In addition to its role in SIBO, excessive hydrogen sulfide is a possible cause of ulcerative colitis and colon cancer (Medani M, 2011.) When present in normal levels, hydrogen sulfide has protective functions (Elsheikh W, 2014).

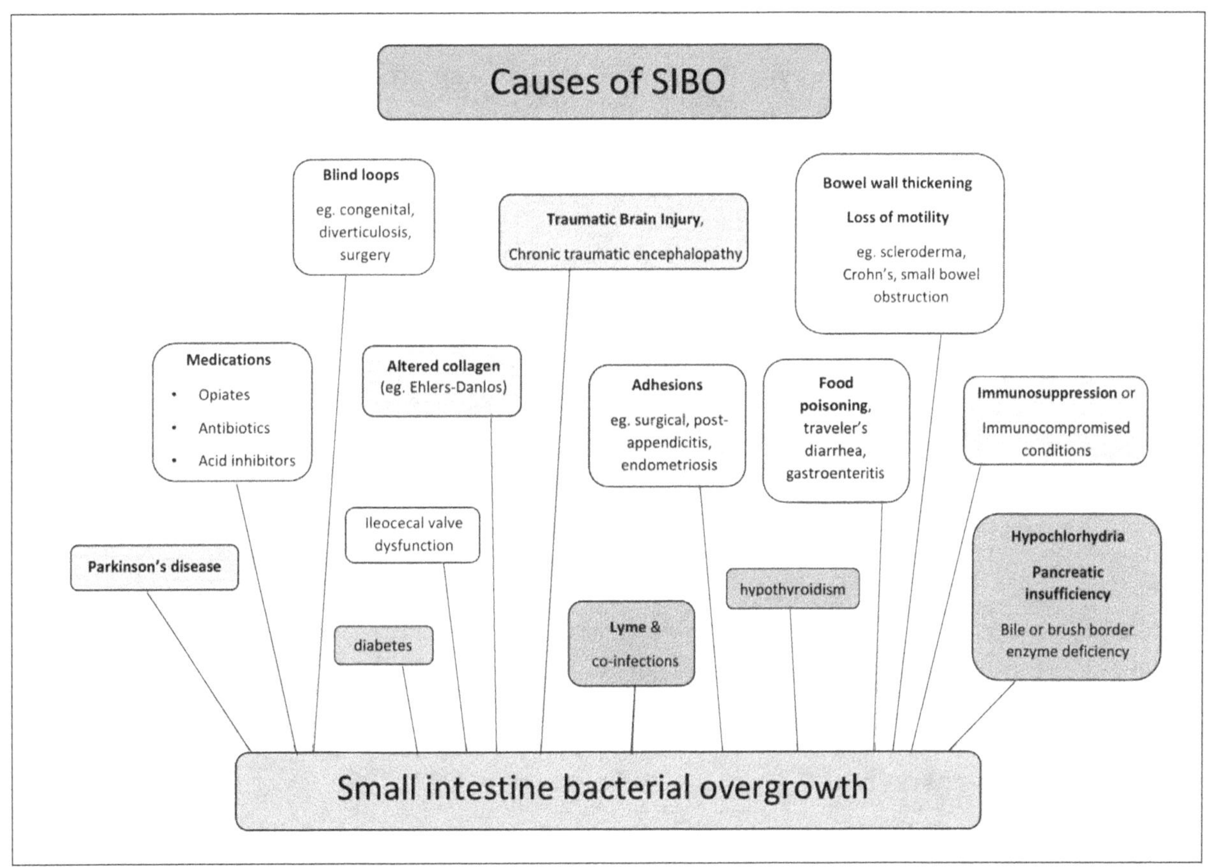

Fig. 16.1. Underlying causes for SIBO and IMO.

UNDERLYING CAUSES FOR SIBO AND IMO

A key to preventing recurrence of SIBO and IMO is to uncover and treat the underlying causes (when possible).

Both patients and physicians often ask whether SIBO and IMO are curable. Many times, a course marked by frequent recurrences and serial treatment regimens is needed. The key is to uncover the predisposing cause(s). When the underlying cause can be removed or at least controlled, relapsing SIBO/IMO can be cured or greatly reduced. In other cases, SIBO/IMO may be a chronic condition that requires ongoing management. The good news is that there are many options for control and treatment which will be discussed below.

Key Underlying Causes Can Produce These Results

- alter the structure or function of **collagen**

- alter the tone of the **ileocecal valve**

- elevate tissue glucose levels

- decrease immune function
- create intestinal **blind loops**

- create intestinal compression or obstruction (thickening of the bowel wall or adhesion/**stricture** formation)

- decrease migrating motor complex activity (Siebecker A, Sandberg-Lewis S, 2013)

Trauma and Lifestyle Factors That May Trigger SIBO/IMO

- traumatic brain injury

- alcohol consumption

- medication use (opiates, antispasmodics, anticholinergics, immune suppressants, etc.)

- physical overtraining

As discussed in chapter eight—*Treatment: Reduce CARBS; Relieve Reflux*, people who consume or engage in behaviors included in the mnemonic C.A.R.B.S. are at an increased risk for reflux disease.

Altered Collagen—Hypermobile Ehlers-Danlos Syndrome (hEDS)

Ehlers-Danlos syndrome is a group of thirteen disorders which includes the hypermobile type. The hypermobile EDS type is the most common of these **collagen variants** (https://www. ehlers-danlos.com/is-eds-rare-or-common/). The guidelines now also include the terms Hypermobility Spectrum Disorder as well as hypermobile EDS. When the data on both these conditions is combined, the estimated incidence rate is between 1 in 600 and 1 in 900 persons. The other genetic forms of EDS are rare or ultrarare.   Joint hypermobility is associated with a higher risk of reflux disease. To determine the presence of hEDS, the Beighton score, a nine point physical test, is used. Joint hypermobility is

Hiatal hernia and GERD are common in hypermobility syndrome.

rated at the knees, elbows, first and fifth finger joints, and lumbar spine (see http://www.ehlers-danlos.org/about-eds/getting-a-diagnosis/beighton-score/). Excessive stretch marks or scars, easy bruising and bleeding, soft-velvety or abnormally elastic skin, chronic joint and limb pain, recurrent joint **subluxations** or dislocations and fatigue are other common manifestations.

Gastrointestinal manifestations of hEDS include hiatal hernia, GERD, abdominal wall and inguinal hernias, **colonic redundancy** and **prolapse**, anal prolapse, celiac disease, **delayed gastric emptying** and ileocecal valve dysfunction. GERD occurs in 68% of hEDS patients (Zeitoun JD, 2013). The reflux in these patients is often resistant to standard treatments.

hEDS patients are often prone to acute and chronic joint, muscle and tendon pain which may lead to greater use of narcotic pain medicines, additionally triggering SIBO/IMO due to slowing of the MMC. The prolapse and kinks in the small intestine may also slow down the MMC.

In a Swedish **whole population-based study** (28,631 subjects) the incidence of celiac disease was increased by 49% in hEDS (Laszkowska M, 2016). An Argentinian study found that 30.1% of undiagnosed celiac disease patients had moderate to severe GERD compared to only 5.7% of those without a celiac diagnosis. Starting a gluten-free diet brought rapid and lasting relief from GERD symptoms for a significant number of these newly diagnosed celiac patients (Nachman F et al, 2011).

ALTERED ILEOCECAL VALVE FUNCTION

A properly functioning ileocecal valve prevents **cecoileal** reflux. The colon typically contains 100 billion bacteria per milliliter of stool compared to a thousand bacteria per milliliter in the small intestine. Therefore, reflux from the cecum through this valve may introduce huge numbers of organisms into the ileum. If the migrating motor complex or other compensatory contractions cannot override this reflux, SIBO is likely. In a **retrospective study** of 23 subjects, ileocecal valve pressure (muscle tone of the valve) was significantly lower in those with a positive lactulose SIBO breath test compared to a negative test (Rowland BC, 2014).

ELEVATED BLOOD SUGAR AND DIABETIC ENTEROPATHY

SIBO/IMO incidence is significantly higher in patients with

increased abdominal fat, **metabolic syndrome**, and type 2 diabetes mellitus (Fialho A, 2016). Type 1 diabetes mellitus is associated with significantly higher rates of SIBO when intestinal nerve function has been damaged by persistently high blood sugar levels (Ojetti V, 2009). The term for this intestinal nerve dysfunction is **autonomic neuropathy.**

Gastroparesis, pancreatitis, and **non-alcoholic fatty liver disease** (NAFLD) are all diabetes associated complications. SIBO is reported to be "very common" in patients with gastroparesis who have symptoms of abdominal pain and bloating. This is especially true for those who have a greater than a five-year history of gastroparesis (Reddymasu SC, 2010). A **meta-analysis** of chronic pancreatitis found that one third of people with this diagnosis have SIBO which is significantly increased compared to people who have never suffered from pancreatitis. Looking only at studies that employed lactulose as a test substrate (rather than glucose) showed 73.3% had SIBO/IMO. The successful treatment of SIBO was associated with clinical improvement (Capurso G, 2016). In a case control study of 372 subjects, NAFLD was over twice as likely in SIBO/IMO positive patients compared to a control group (Fialho A, 2016).

Tight blood glucose control in diabetics is essential to prevent chronic relapsing SIBO/IMO.

Immunocompromised States

There is evidence that HIV/AIDS, **IgA deficiency,** and **common variable immunodeficiency** are associated with SIBO/IMO. Bacterial overgrowth may be one more example of the opportunistic infections that these patients may develop (Bures J, 2010). In the case of HIV/AIDS the mechanism may be related to **hypochlorhydria** (Lake-Bakaar G, 1988).

Blind Loops

Non-draining pockets of small intestine allow decreased clearance and increased growth of microorganisms (Rana SV, 2008). Bariatric surgery such as Roux-en-Y (Dolan RD, 2021) and congenital anomalies such as **duodenal duplication** and **small intestine diverticula** foster overgrowth as well (Mathias JR, 1985).

Intestinal Compression

An uncommon cause of complete or partial obstruction of the

upper small bowel is superior mesenteric artery (SMA) syndrome. I have seen several cases in which SMA syndrome caused recurrent SIBO. Rapid weight loss, abdominal trauma, aortic aneurysm repair or spinal surgery (especially surgery to correct scoliosis) may cause a silent SMA syndrome to become symptomatic (Naseem Z, 2015). SMA syndrome is most often diagnosed by an upper GI barium series or abdominal CT (Kaur A, 2016).

BOWEL WALL THICKENING

Scleroderma has a strong association with SIBO/IMO because thickened collagen deposition stiffens the small bowel and the esophagus, leading to decreased motility. This makes esophageal reflux and SIBO more likely. "CREST syndrome" is a modified form of scleroderma in which the "E" stands for esophageal dysmotility, a frequent cause of reflux in these cases.

ADHESIONS AND STRICTURES

Bands of scar tissue can form in response to injury, radiation, surgery, some infections, internal bleeding, or inflammation. Such bands are called **adhesions** (Liakakos T, 2001). **Strictures** are scar-like bands that develop on the inner lining of digestive organs, narrowing the opening. Both adhesions and strictures slow motility and frequently cause microorganism overgrowth.

TRAUMATIC BRAIN INJURY (TBI)

One of the factors that appears to trigger dysmotility and therefore some cases of SIBO is traumatic brain injury. At one end of the spectrum a patient may have had severe trauma with coma prior to the onset of digestive problems. At the other extreme, there may have been little or no direct impact to the skull, just a shaking of the brain inside the skull. To uncover these types of traumas the physician must understand that "shaking of the brain" within the rigid cranium is the key issue. "Heading" the ball in soccer, whiplash injuries, proximity to explosions (such as military personnel exposed to improvised explosive device blasts), shaken baby syndrome and other injuries can all lead to motility changes in the gut. Reflux is a common cause of symptoms in patients with brain damage. The LES pressure of cats was measured before and after exposure to modest increases in **intracranial pressure.** Under higher pressure, which simulates the brain changes in TBI, the LES pressure dropped by nearly two-thirds (Vane DW, 1982). This GERD promoting effect lasted for at least six weeks.

ALCOHOL CONSUMPTION

Heavy drinking and alcoholism, as well as moderate use of alcohol, is significantly associated with increased SIBO risk (Gabbard SL, 2014). In a retrospective review of 210 patients who had lactulose breath testing, moderate consumption of alcohol (1 drink per day for women and 2 drinks per day for men) was a strong risk factor for SIBO/IMO. Alcohol consumption is a risk factor for reflux and esophageal cancer.

MEDICATION USE

A meta-analysis of studies using duodenal cultures as a diagnostic tool concluded that PPI use statistically increased SIBO risk (Lo WK, 2013). This effect was not found using glucose breath testing and they didn't include research using lactulose breath tests.

HOW SIBO AND IMO CAUSE REFLUX

Bacterial fermentation produces hydrogen and/or hydrogen sulfide gas. In addition, archaeal organisms produce methane (Kim G, 2012). The quantity of gas may be extensive, causing severe bloating and distention (Youn YH 2011). Excess gas can then exit the body as flatulence or belching. A portion is also absorbed into the blood and eventually filters through the lungs to exit on exhalation. Excess methane slows gut motility. The pressure created by any of these gases increases intra-abdominal pressure (Kim KM, 2012).

DIAGNOSIS OF SIBO AND IMO

As I've mentioned, hydrogen/methane breath testing is the most common method of assessing SIBO. Instrumentation is available from the Quintron Instrument Company in Milwaukee, Wisconsin. Quintron builds and distributes the Breathtracker, used to measure hydrogen and methane after the patient eats a prep diet for one to two days, followed by an overnight fast. After collection of the fasting baseline specimen, a solution of lactulose—a synthetic sugar—is ingested. Lactulose is used because most bacteria, but not humans, produce the enzymes to digest it. Transit time for lactulose through the stomach and small bowel is 90 - 120 minutes. Breath may be sampled and immediately analysed at a lab, or these samples may be acquired at home using a series of tubes to be sent to a lab for later analysis. Testing for methane in addition to hydrogen is important because treatment varies based on the type of gas. One U.S. lab also offers a test that measures all 3 gases, methane, hydrogen and hydrogen sulfide.

Preparation for the test varies from lab to lab, but a typical prep diet is limited to white rice, fish/poultry/meat, eggs, hard cheeses, clear beef or chicken broth (not bone broth or bouillon), oil, salt, and pepper. The purpose of the prep diet is to get a clear reaction to the lactulose or glucose solution by eliminating fermentable foods prior to testing. In cases of constipation, two days of prep diet may be needed to adequately reduce baseline gases. Antibiotics should not be used for at least two weeks prior to an initial test although some sources recommend avoiding them for four weeks (Eisenmann, 2008.) Laxatives, including high dose magnesium and/or vitamin C, should be avoided for at least four days prior to the day of the test. This is especially important if these laxatives cause loose or liquid stools which may lead to falsely low gas levels. If symptoms allow, proton pump inhibitors should also be eliminated for at least seven days before testing (Costa MB, 2012.)

For more detailed information on testing and interpretation of results, consult my textbook, *Functional Gastroenterology*, second edition, 2017.

TREATMENT OF SIBO AND IMO

In 2006, Dr. Pimentel shared his treatment algorithm for SIBO which included the use of prescription antibiotics or elemental diet (Pimentel M, 2006).   The approach Dr. Allison Siebecker and I devised over the last twelve years offers two additional options: diet and herbal antibiotics (See SIBO/IMO Treatment Algorithm below). These options should be chosen and supervised under the care of a healthcare provider.

HERBAL ANTIBIOTICS

While there have been only two published reports of successful herbal treatment of SIBO (Logan A, 2002 and Chedid V, 2014), my experience is that they have similar effectiveness to pharmaceutical antibiotics. Chedid et al studied patients with SIBO using a positive lactulose breath test. A negative breath test after treatment was seen in 34% of the rifaximin or a multiple prescription antibiotic treated group vs. 46% of the herbal treated group.

The typical prescription treatment for hydrogen SIBO is rifaximin (brand name Xifaxan). Standard prescription for methane

IMO is a combination of rifaximin with either neomycin or metronidazole.

My approach to herbal treatment for hydrogen SIBO is either berberine containing herbs such as goldenseal (*Hydrastis canadensis*), Oregon grape (*Berberis aquafolium*) and amur corktree (*Phellodendron amurense*) or emulsified oregano extract (*Origanum vulgare*).

For methane IMO, I use allicin extract (a fructan-free extract of garlic), emulsified oregano, or a combination of quebracho (*Quebracho colorado*), horse chestnut (*Aesculus hippocastanum*), and peppermint (*Mentha haplocalyx*). The latter three are found in the product brand named Atrantil.

For more detailed information on treatment, please refer to Chapter Eight in my textbook, *Functional Gastroenterology,* or for a general overview see my webinar/lecture at https://hmmpdx. com/videos "How to Help Your Doctor Treat Your SIBO".

Probiotics

Three preliminary studies have investigated the use of probiotics alone or combined with prescription antibiotics for the treatment of SIBO. In the first, six bacterial species were used: *Bifidobacterium bifidum, Bifidobacterium lactis, Bifidobacterium longum, Lactobacillus acidophilu*s, *Lactobacillus rhamnosus,* and *Streptococcus thermophilus* (Kwak DS, 2014). This combination significantly normalized the breath test and alleviated symptoms while a single strain of *Lactobacillus fermentum* (Stotzer PO,1996) did not. A third study, which was found to have significant benefits for normalizing the breath test and relieving abdominal pain, flatulence, belching, and diarrhea, used probiotic *Bacillus coagulans* spores following prescription antibiotic treatment (Khalighi AR, 2014).

Diet

The nutrition plan I use most often to reduce symptoms and recurrence of SIBO/IMO after treatment is the SIBO Specific Foodguide. This is a combination of the Specific Carbohydrate Diet, the low FODMAP diet and the clinical experience of Dr. Siebecker in her treatment of SIBO with diet. Bacteria use carbohydrates as their energy source and ferment them, creating gases. A low carbohydrate diet can directly reduce symptoms by decreasing

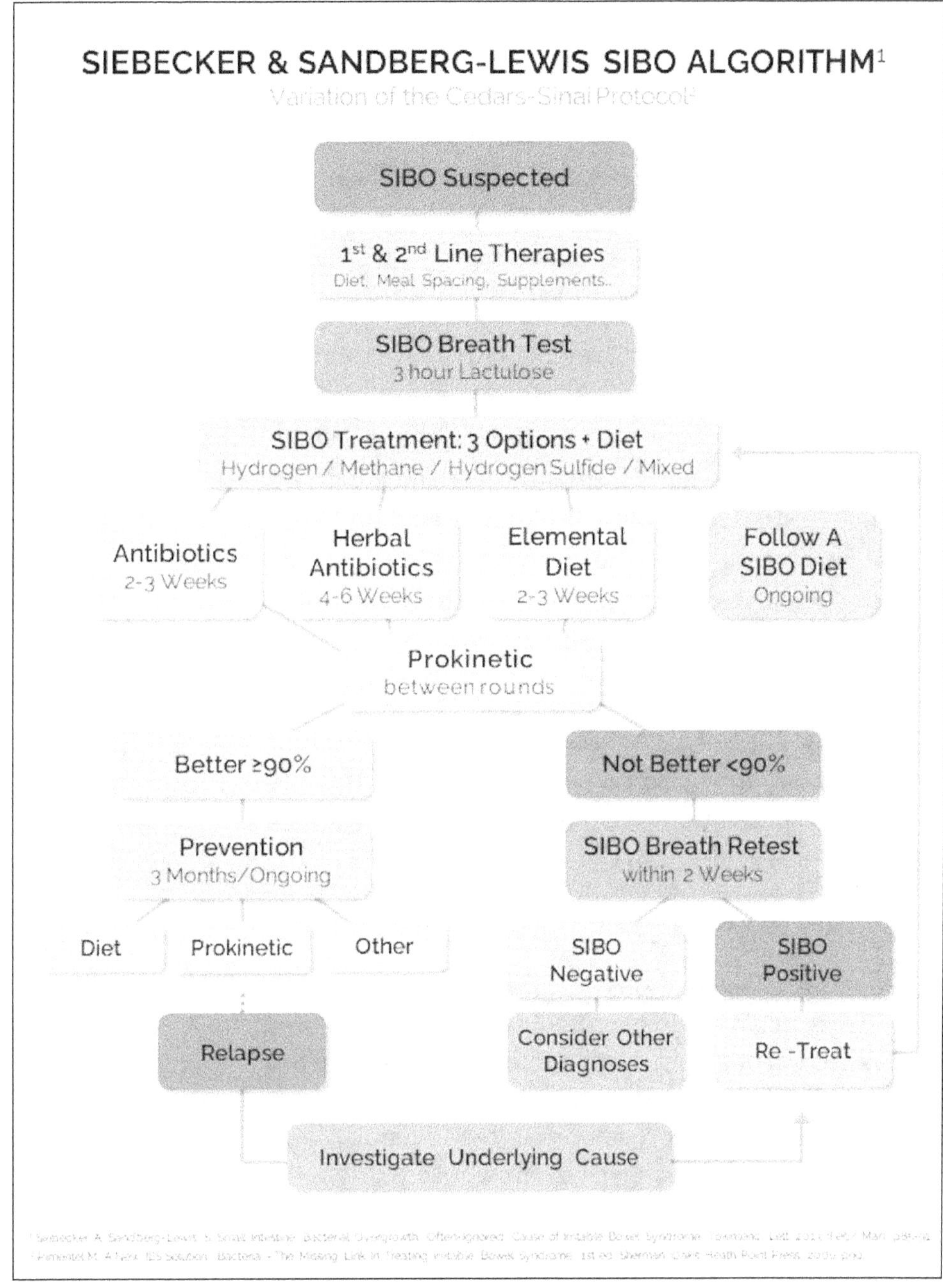

Fig. 16.2. The Siebecker and Sandberg-Lewis SIBO treatment protocol.

the amount of gas produced (Ong DK, 2010). Reducing carbohydrates may also decrease the overall microbial load, though formal studies to validate this are lacking. See chapter nine for more details on this and other diets for reflux and bacterial overgrowth.

ELEMENTAL DIET

An elemental diet can be used in place of prescription or herbal antibiotics to rapidly decrease overgrowth. In the treatment of SIBO/IMO, elemental diet is used to the exclusion of all other food sources. These products are a powdered mix of free form amino acids, fat, vitamins, and minerals as well as rapidly absorbed carbohydrates. The concept behind this treatment is that the nutrients will be absorbed before reaching the bacteria, thus feeding the patient but starving the flora. It is used in place of all meals, for two to three weeks, and has a success rate of 80-85% (Pimentel M, 2004) At the time of this writing the only published study used the Nestle product Vivonex® Plus.

Patients should be warned that Vivonex® Plus or homemade elemental diets taste bitter. Healthier, more pleasant tasting versions of elemental formulae are also available. These include Integrative Therapeutics' Physicians' Elemental Diet and Functional Medicine Formulations' Elemental Heal. Before deciding to follow an elemental diet, please watch the three videos by Dr. Allison Siebecker at https://www.siboinfo.com/elemental-formula, which explain the process and cautions in detail.

IMPORTANT: Underweight patients must be sure to take the full recommended number of daily servings to prevent weight loss. Elemental formulas may also be used as "safe" foods while traveling or ingested in addition to other foods to add calories and nutrients to highly restricted diets.

PREVENTION OF SIBO RECURRENCE

Prevention of SIBO recurrence should always follow treatment. The prevention stage includes a low fermentation diet as well as a nightly prokinetic herbal or prescription medicine to enhance the cleansing function of the migrating motor complex. Examples of prescription prokinetics include prucalopride (brand name Motegrity or Resolor), low dose erythromycin or low dose naltrexone. Herbal options include ginger root, ginger and artichoke (brand name Motility Activator), a German liquid herbal combination featuring *Iberis amara* (brand name Iberogast) and a combination of ginger, 5HTP, vitamin B6, and acetyl–L–carnitine (brand name Motilpro).

A few years ago, I asked my son to help me answer in a graphic format the many questions patients have regarding SIBO. It's a complicated subject, so we aimed for an overview of several main points. The result was a patient handout we called ***Nothin' Funnies About Small Intestine Bacterial Overgrowth,*** which is presented here for your enjoyment. 

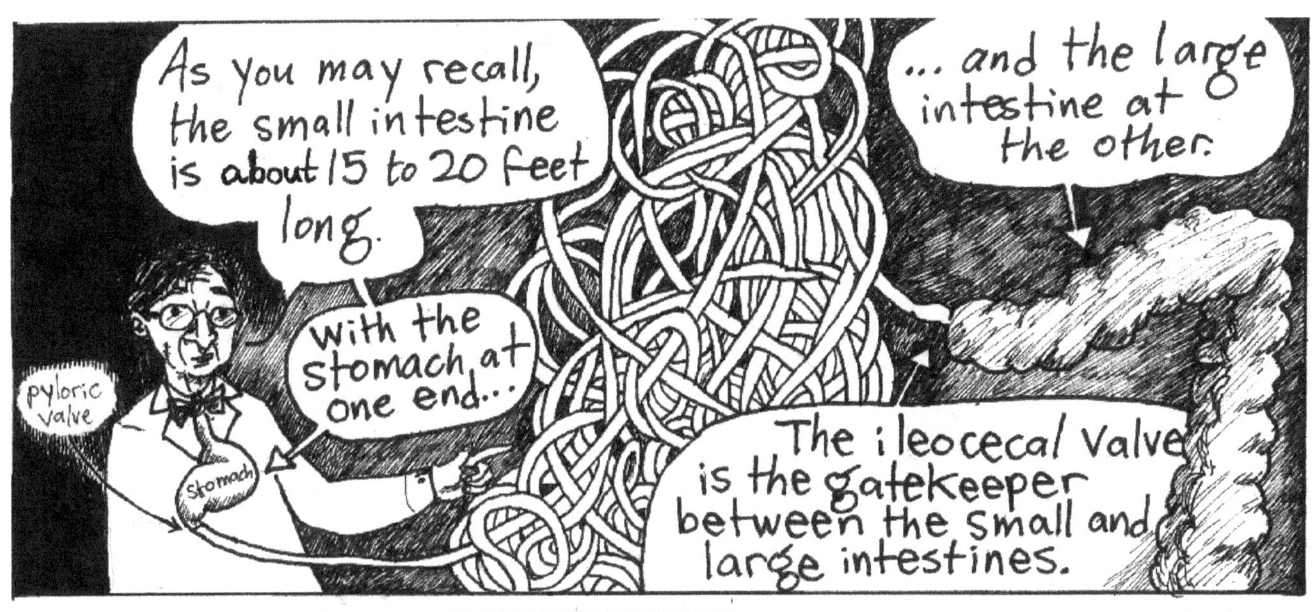
As you may recall, the small intestine is about 15 to 20 feet long.
With the stomach at one end...
pyloric valve
Stomach
... and the large intestine at the other.
The ileocecal valve is the gatekeeper between the small and large intestines.

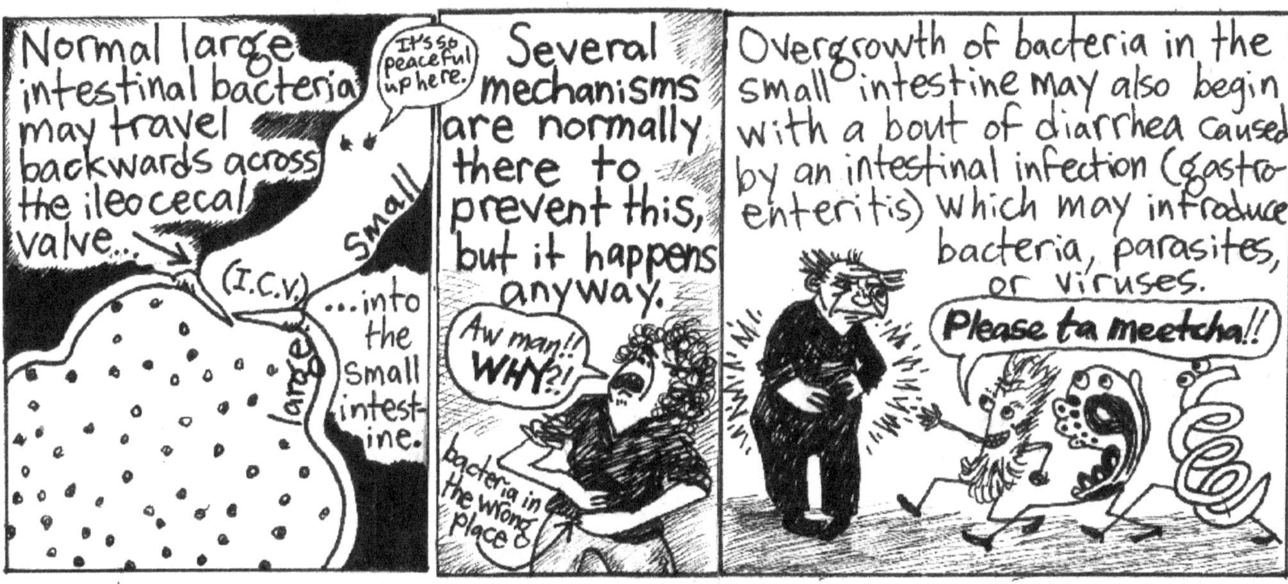
Normal large intestinal bacteria may travel backwards across the ileocecal valve...
It's so peaceful up here.
(I.C.V.)
Small
large
...into the small intest- ine.
Several mechanisms are normally there to prevent this, but it happens anyway.
Aw man!! WHY?!
bacteria in the wrong place
Overgrowth of bacteria in the small intestine may also begin with a bout of diarrhea caused by an intestinal infection (gastro- enteritis) which may introduce bacteria, parasites, or viruses.
MII
Please ta meetcha!!

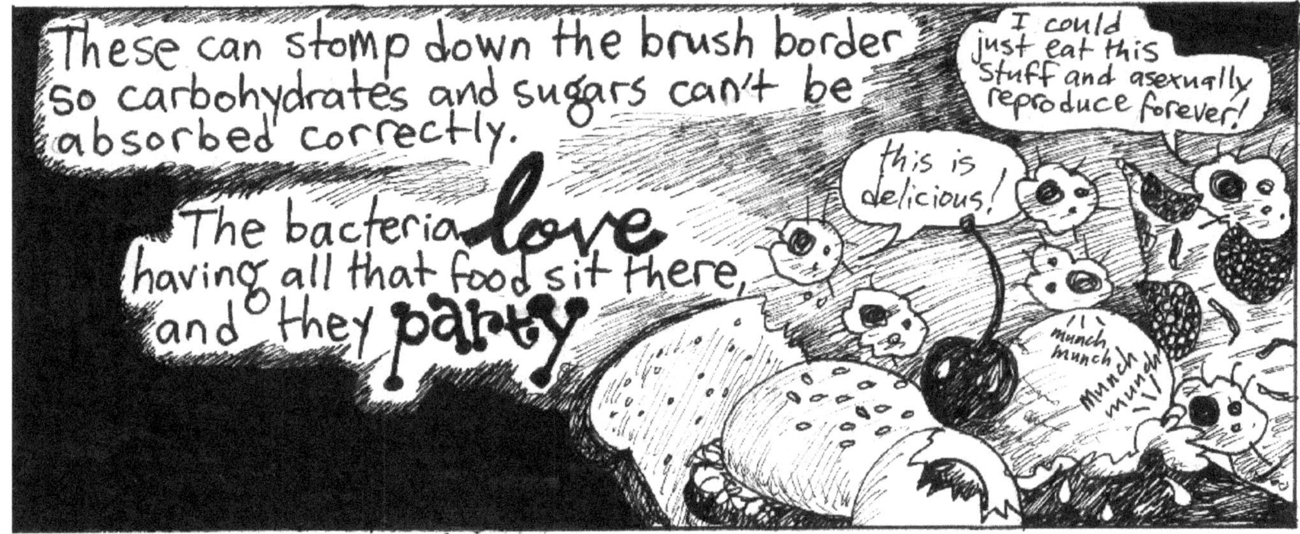
These can stomp down the brush border so carbohydrates and sugars can't be absorbed correctly.
The bacteria love having all that food sit there, and they party
I could just eat this stuff and asexually reproduce forever!
this is delicious!
munch munch
munch munch

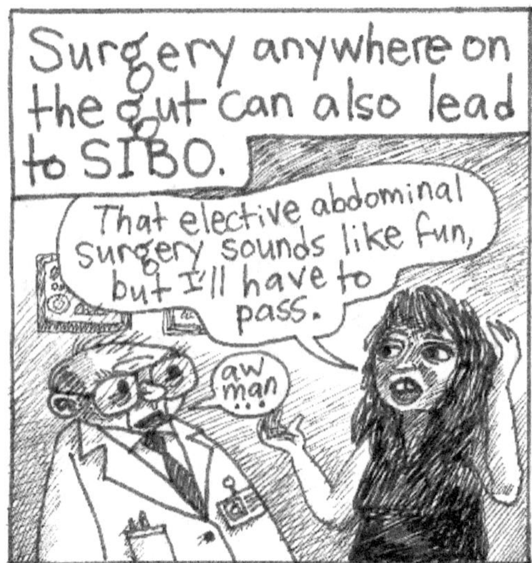
Surgery anywhere on the gut can also lead to SIBO.
That elective abdominal surgery sounds like fun, but I'll have to pass.
aw man

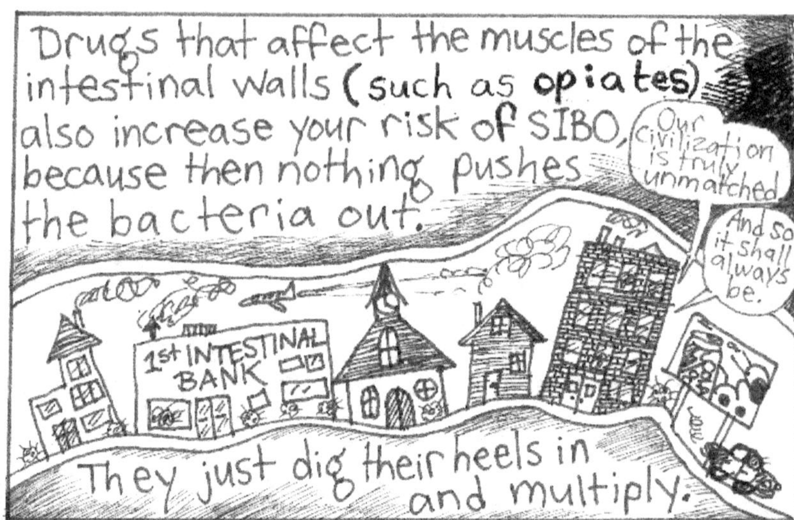
Drugs that affect the muscles of the intestinal walls (such as opiates) also increase your risk of SIBO, because then nothing pushes the bacteria out.
Our civilization is truly unmatched
And so it shall always be.
1st INTESTINAL BANK
They just dig their heels in and multiply.

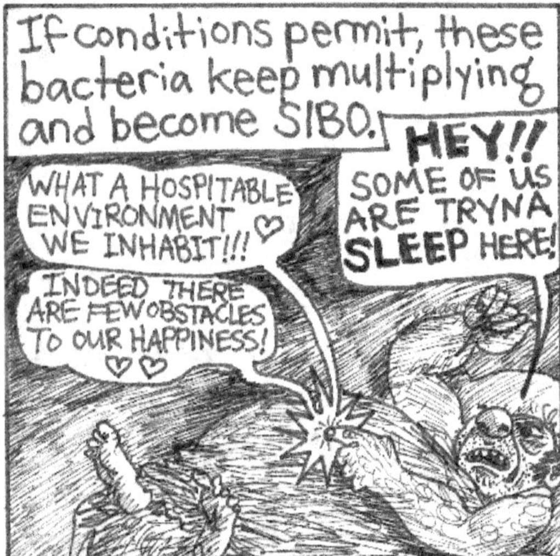
If conditions permit, these bacteria keep multiplying and become SIBO.
WHAT A HOSPITABLE ENVIRONMENT WE INHABIT!!!
INDEED THERE ARE FEW OBSTACLES TO OUR HAPPINESS!
HEY!! SOME OF US ARE TRYNA SLEEP HERE!

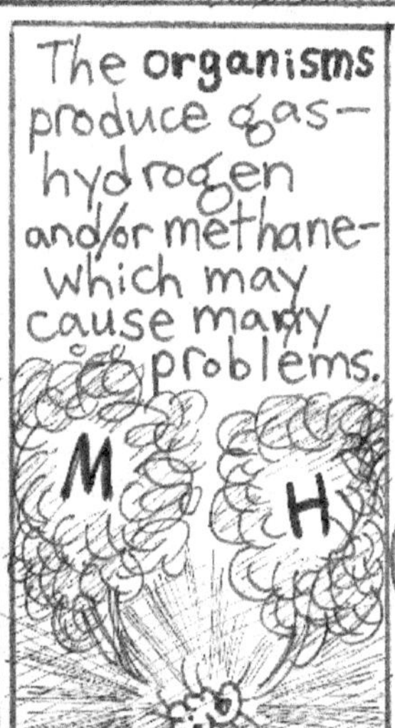
The organisms produce gas— hydrogen and/or methane— which may cause many problems.
M   H

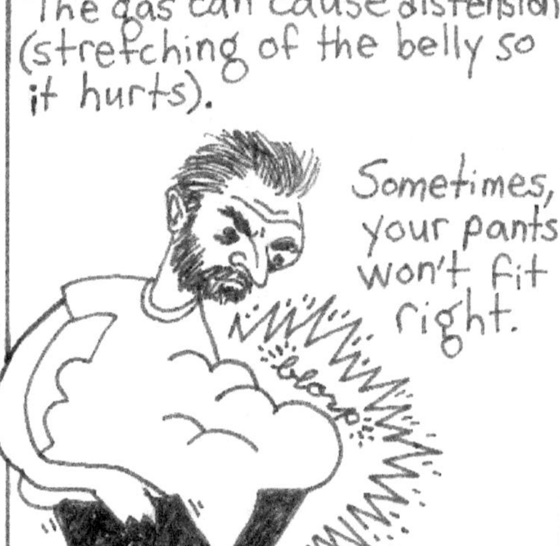
The gas can cause distension (stretching of the belly so it hurts).
Sometimes, your pants won't fit right.

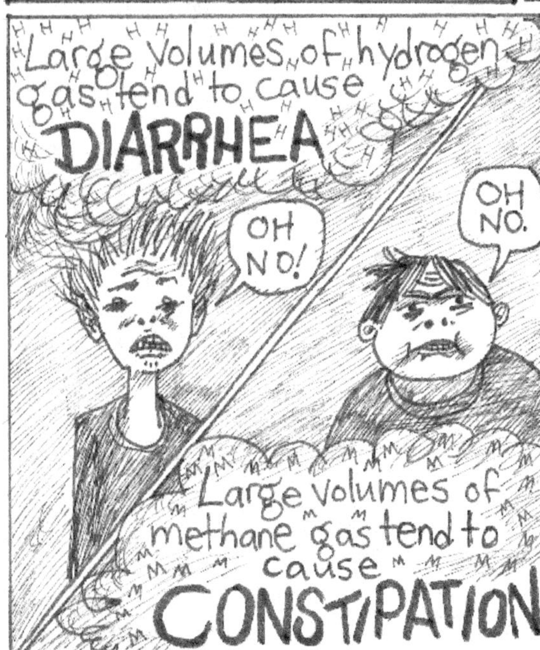
Large volumes of hydrogen gas tend to cause DIARRHEA
OH NO!
OH NO.
Large volumes of methane gas tend to cause CONSTIPATION

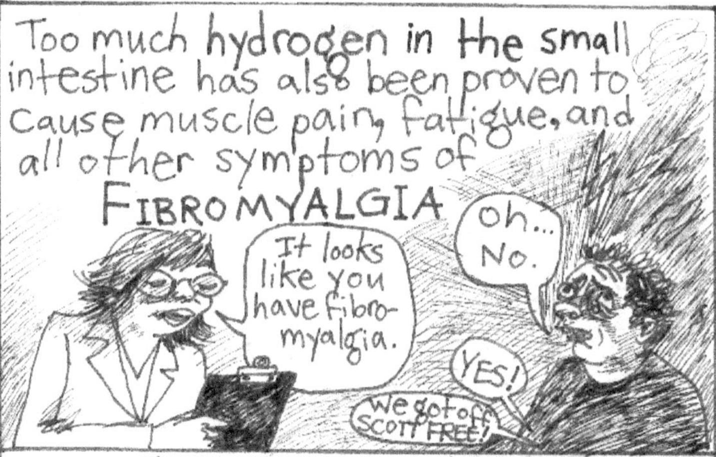
Too much hydrogen in the small intestine has also been proven to cause muscle pain, fatigue, and all other symptoms of FIBROMYALGIA
It looks like you have fibromyalgia.
Oh... No.
YES!
We got off scott FREE!
Your doctor may mistakenly diagnose fibromyalgia on the basis of these symptoms, in which case you'll get meds that just suppress the symptoms while the SIBO worsens, undetected.

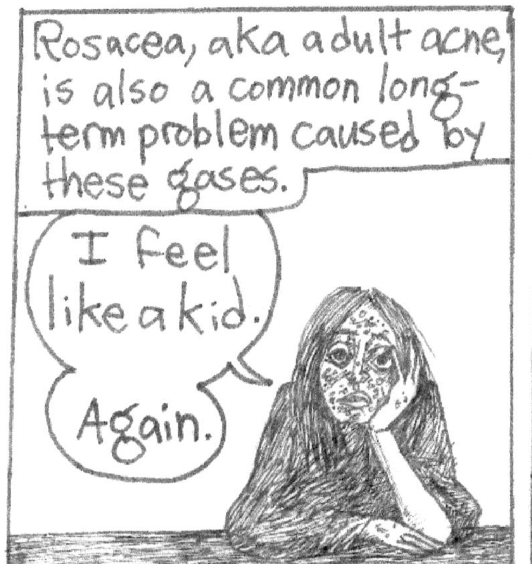
Rosacea, aka adult acne, is also a common long-term problem caused by these gases.
I feel like a kid.
Again.

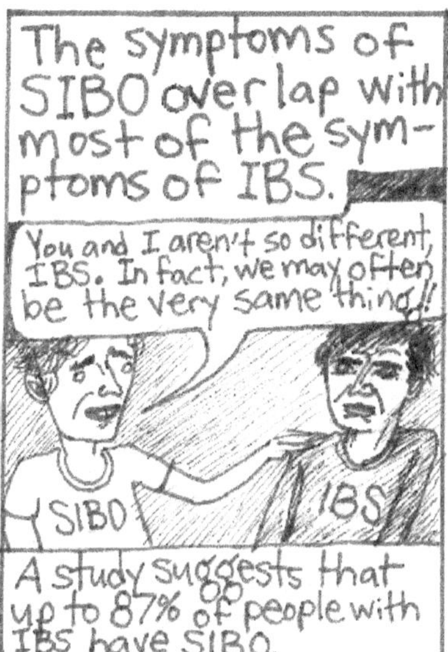
The symptoms of SIBO overlap with most of the symptoms of IBS.
You and I aren't so different, IBS. In fact, we may often be the very same thing!!
SIBO
IBS
A study suggests that up to 87% of people with IBS have SIBO.

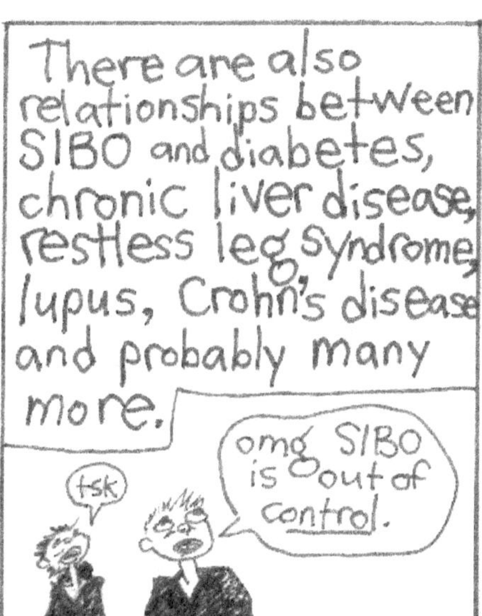
There are also relationships between SIBO and diabetes, chronic liver disease, restless leg syndrome, lupus, Crohn's disease and probably many more.
tsk
omg SIBO is out of control.

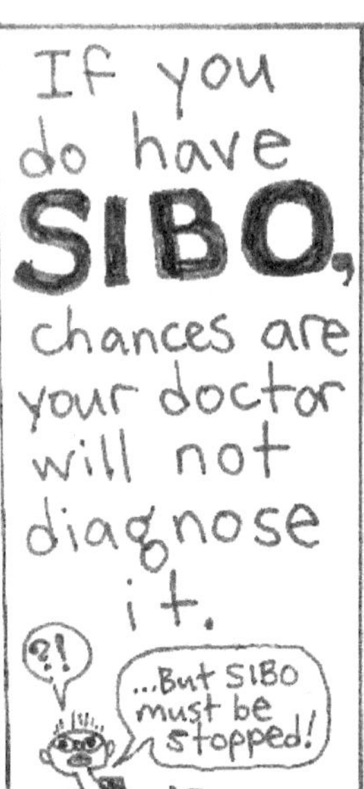
If you do have SIBO, chances are your doctor will not diagnose it.
?!
...But SIBO must be stopped!

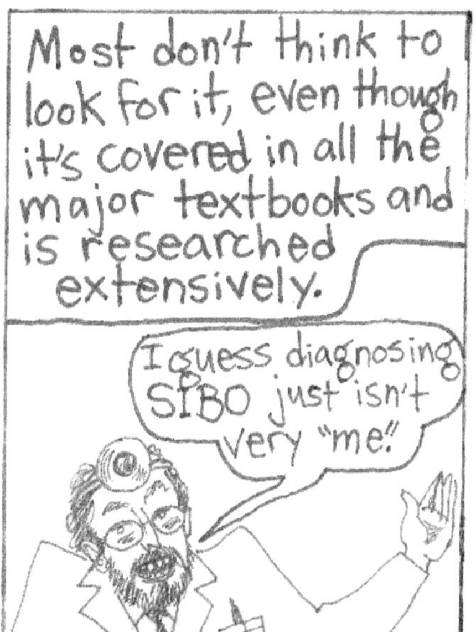
Most don't think to look for it, even though it's covered in all the major textbooks and is researched extensively.
I guess diagnosing SIBO just isn't very "me!"

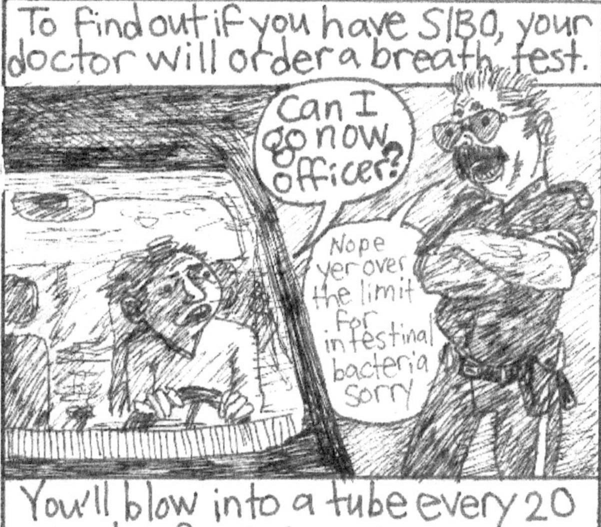
To find out if you have SIBO, your doctor will order a breath test.
Can I go now officer?
Nope yer over the limit for intestinal bacteria sorry
You'll blow into a tube every 20 minutes for 2 to 3 hours.

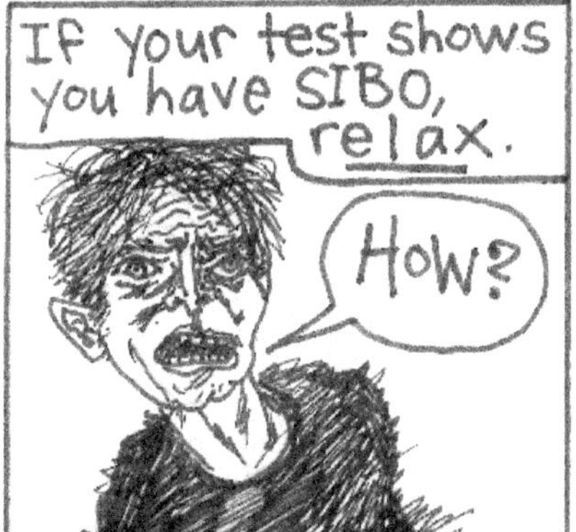
If your test shows you have SIBO, relax.
How?
There are effective treatments for this problem.

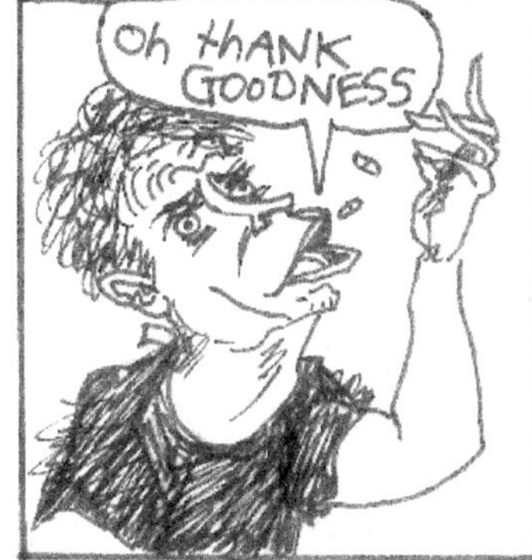
Treatment starts with one or sometimes 2 antibiotics for about 10 days.
Oh thANK GOODNESS

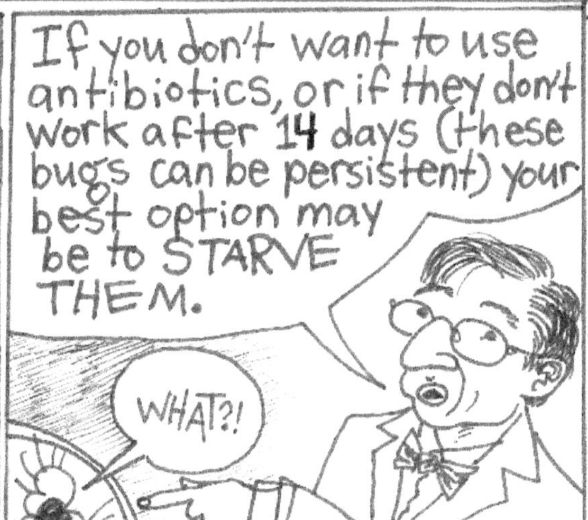
If you don't want to use antibiotics, or if they don't work after 14 days (these bugs can be persistent) your best option may be to STARVE THEM.
WHAT?!

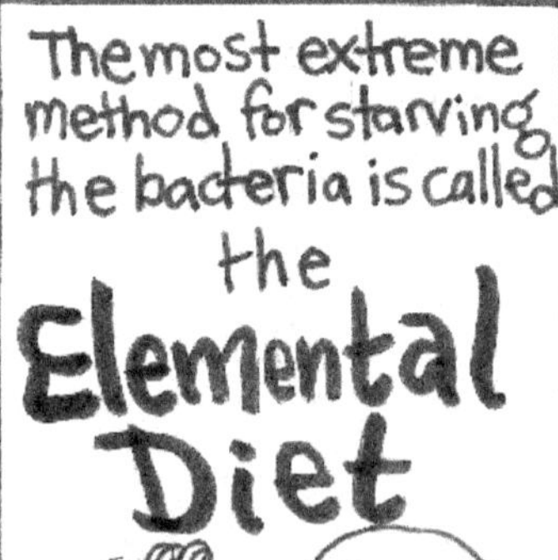

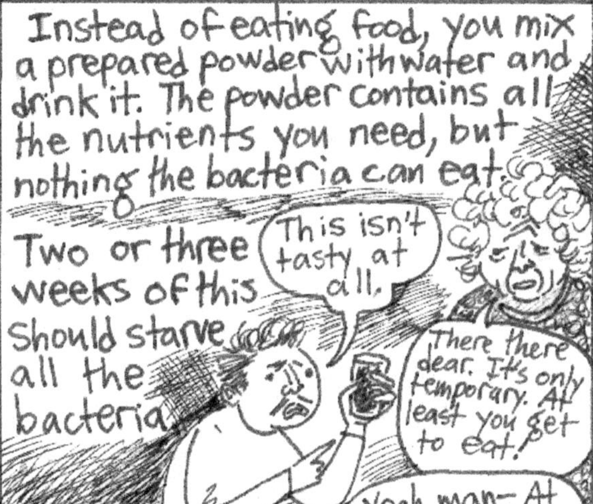

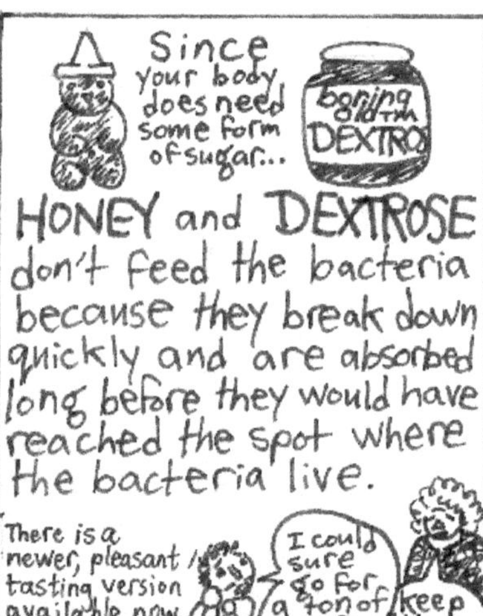

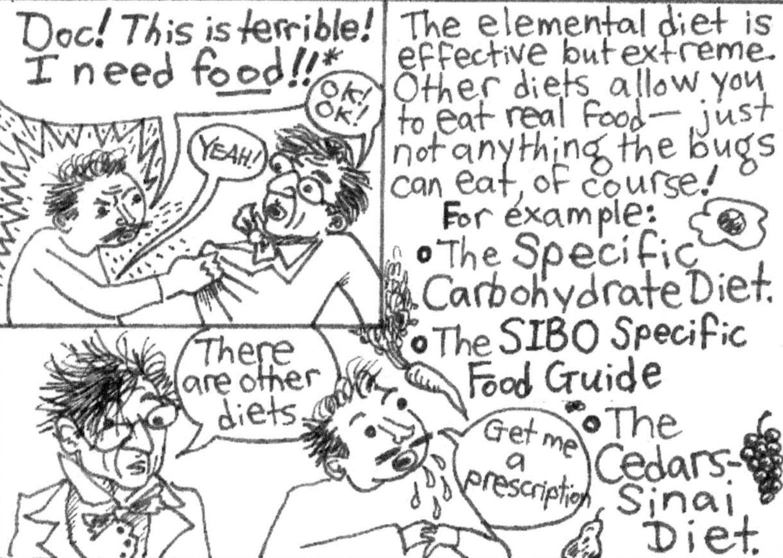

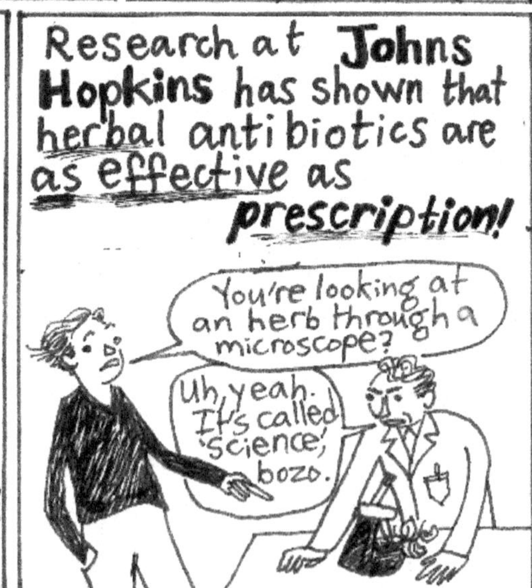

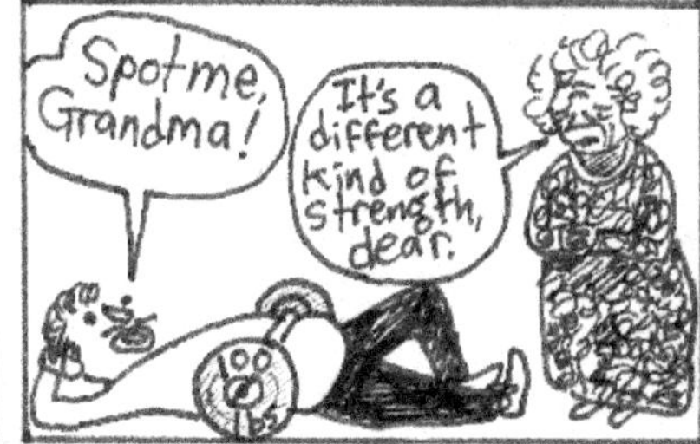

Making sure there is enough **Stomach acid, pancreatic enzymes,** and **bile** in your system will help prevent recurrence of the bacterial overgrowth.

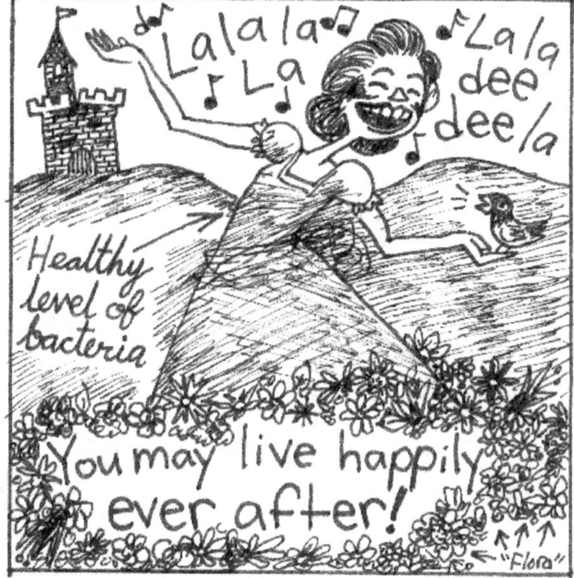

*Please don't treat your doctor like this.

CITATIONS

Peralta S et al, Small intestine bacterial overgrowth and irritable bowel syndrome-related symptoms: experience with Rifaximin. World J Gastroenterol. 2009 Jun 7;15(21):2628-31. PMID: 19496193

Lin HC, et al. Small intestinal bacterial overgrowth: a framework for understanding irritable bowel syndrome. JAMA. 2004 Aug 18;292(7):852-8. PMID: 15316000

Pyleris E et al, The prevalence of overgrowth by aerobic bacteria in the small intestine by small bowel culture: relationship with irritable bowel syndrome. Dig Dis Sci. 2012 May;57(5):1321-9. PMID: 22262197

Pimentel M, Chow EJ, Lin HC, Normalization of lactulose breath testing correlates with symptom improvement in irritable bowel syndrome. A double-blind, randomized, placebo-controlled study. Am J Gastroenterol. 2003 Feb;98(2):412-9. PMID: 12591062

Haworth JJ, Boyle N, Vales A, Hobson AR, The prevalence of intestinal dysbiosis in patients referred for antireflux surgery. Surg Endosc. 2021 Dec;35(12):7112-7119. PMID: 33475845

Jacobs C Adame EC, Attaluri A, Valestin J et al, Dysmotility and proton pump inhibitor use are independent risk factors for small intestinal bacterial and/or fungal overgrowth. Aliment Pharmacol Ther. 2013;37(11):1103–1111. PMID: 23574267

Imhann F, Bonder MJ, Vich Vila A, Fu J, et al. Proton pump inhibitors affect the gut microbiome. Gut. 2016;65(5):740. PMID: 26657899

Anantharaju A, Klamut M, Small intestinal bacterial overgrowth: a possible risk factor for metabolic bone disease. Nutr Rev. 2003 Apr;61(4):132-5. PMID: 12795446

Kim KM, Kim B-T, Lee D-J, Park S-B et al. Erosive esophagitis may be related to small intestinal bacterial overgrowth. Scand J Gastroenterol. 2012 May;47(5):493-8. PMID: 22416969

Lauritano EC, Bilotta AL, Gabrielli M, Scarpellini E, et al. Association between hypothyroidism and small intestinal bacterial overgrowth. J Clin Endocrinol Metab. 2007 Nov;92(11):4180-4. PMID: 17698907

Almeida JA, Kim R, Stoita A, McIver CJ, et al, Lactose malabsorption in the elderly: role of small intestinal bacterial overgrowth. Scand J Gastroenterol. 2008;43(2):146-54. PMID: 18224561

Kaur J, Rana SV, Gupta R, Gupta V et al. Prolonged orocecal transit time enhances serum bile acids through bacterial overgrowth, contributing factor to gallstone disease. J Clin Gastroenterol. 2014 Apr;48(4):365-9. PMID: 24598592

Klaus J, Spaniol U, Adler U, Mason RA et al. Small intestinal bacterial overgrowth mimicking acute flare as a pitfall in patients with Crohn's Disease. BMC Gastroenterol. 2009 Jul 30;9:61. PMID: 19643023

Marie I, Ducrotté P, Denis P, Menard JF et al. Small intestinal bacterial overgrowth in systemic sclerosis. Rheumatology (Oxford). 2009 Oct;48(10):1314-9. PMID: 19696066

Rubio-Tapia A, Barton SH, Rosenblatt JE, Murray JA et al. Prevalence of small intestine bacterial overgrowth diagnosed by quantitative culture of intestinal aspirate in celiac disease. J Clin Gastroenterol. 2009 Feb;43(2):157-61. PMID: 18719514

Mancilla A C, Madrid AM, Hurtado C, Orellana C et al. [Small intestine bacterial overgrowth in patients with chronic pancreatitis]. Rev Med Chil. 2008 Aug;136(8):976-80. PMID: 18949180

Tursi A, Brandimarte G, Giorgetti GM, Elisei W et al. Assessment of small intestinal bacterial overgrowth in uncomplicated acute diverticulitis of the colon. World J Gastroenterol. 2005 May 14;11(18):2773-6. PMID: 15884120

Ojetti V, Pitocco D, Scarpellini E, Zaccardi F, et al, Small bowel bacterial overgrowth and type 1 diabetes. Eur Rev Med Pharmacol Sci. 2009 Nov-Dec;13(6):419-23. PMID: 20085122

Goebel A, Buhner S, Schedel R, Lochs H, et al, Altered intestinal permeability in patients with primary fibromyalgia and in patients with complex regional pain syndrome. Rheumatology (Oxford). 2008 Aug;47(8):1223-7. PMID: 18540025

Gupta A, Dhiman RK, Kumari S, Rana S et al, Role of small intestinal bacterial overgrowth and delayed gastrointestinal transit time in cirrhotic patients with minimal hepatic encephalopathy. J Hepatol. 2010 Nov;53(5):849-55. PMID: 20675008

Shanab AA, Scully P, Crosbie O, Buckley M et al, Small intestinal bacterial overgrowth in nonalcoholic steatohepatitis: association with toll-like receptor 4 expression and plasma levels of interleukin 8. Dig Dis Sci. 2011 May;56(5):1524-34. PMID: 21046243

Weinstock LB, Klutke CG, Lin HC, Small intestinal bacterial overgrowth in patients with interstitial cystitis and gastrointestinal symptoms. Dig Dis Sci. 2008 May;53(5):1246-51. PMID: 17932763

Weinstock LB, Walters AS, Restless legs syndrome is associated with irritable bowel syndrome and small intestinal bacterial overgrowth. Sleep Med. 2011 Jun;12(6):610-3. PMID: 21570907

Parodi A, Paolino S, Greco A, Drago F et al, Small intestinal bacterial overgrowth in rosacea: clinical effectiveness of its eradication. Clin Gastroenterol Hepatol. 2008 Jul;6(7):759-64. PMID: 18456568

Fialho A, Fialho A, Schenone A, Thota P et al. Association between small intestinal bacterial overgrowth and deep vein thrombosis. Gastroenterol Rep (Oxf). 2016 Nov;4(4):299-303. PMID: 27044499

Donowitz JR, Haque R, Kirkpatrick BD, Alam M, et al. Small Intestine Bacterial Overgrowth and Environmental Enteropathy in Bangladeshi Children. mBio. 2016 Jan 12;7(1):e02102-15. PMID: 26758185

Pimentel M, Personal communication, 2014

Gabbard SL, Lacy BE, Levine GM, Crowell MD et al. The impact of alcohol consumption and cholecystectomy on small intestinal bacterial overgrowth. Dig Dis Sci. 2014 Mar;59(3):638-44. PMID: 24323179

Jacobs C, Adame EC, Attaluri A, Valestin J et al. Dysmotility and proton pump inhibitor use are independent risk factors for small intestinal bacterial and/or fungal overgrowth. Aliment Pharmacol Ther. 2013 Jun;37(11):1103-11. PMID: 23574267

Takakura W, Pimentel M. Small Intestinal Bacterial Overgrowth and Irritable Bowel Syndrome - An Update. Front Psychiatry. 2020 Jul 10;11:664. PMID: 32754068

Carbonero F, Benefiel AC, Alizadeh-Ghamsari AH, Gaskins HR et al. Microbial pathways in colonic sulfur metabolism and links with health and disease. Front Physiol. 2012 Nov 28;3:448. PMID: 23226130

Million M, Angelakis E, Maraninchi M, Henry M et al. Correlation between body mass index and gut concentrations of Lactobacillus reuteri, Bifidobacterium animalis, Methanobrevibacter smithii and Escherichia coli. Int J Obes (Lond). 2013 Nov;37(11):1460-6. PMID: 23459324

Medani M, Collins D, Docherty NG, Baird AW et al. Emerging role of hydrogen sulfide in colonic physiology and pathophysiology. Inflamm Bowel Dis. 2011 Jul;17(7):1620-5. PMID: 21674719

Elsheikh W, Blackler RW, Flannigan KL, Wallace JL et al. Enhanced chemopreventive effects of a hydrogen sulfide-releasing anti-inflammatory drug (ATB-346) in experimental colorectal cancer. \Nitric Oxide. 2014 Sep 15;41:131-7. PMID: 24747869

Siebecker A, Sandberg-Lewis S, Small Intestine Bacterial Overgrowth: Common but Overlooked Cause of IBS, Nat Doctors News Rev, online Jan 2013.

Zeitoun JD, Lefèvre JH, de Parades V, Séjourné C, et al. Functional digestive symptoms and quality of life in patients with Ehlers-Danlos syndromes: results of a national cohort study on 134 patients. PLoS One. 2013 Nov 22;8(11):e80321. PMID: 24278273

Laszkowska M, Roy A, Lebwohl B, Green PHR et al. Nationwide population-based cohort study of celiac disease and risk of Ehlers-Danlos syndrome and joint hypermobility syndrome. Dig Liver Dis. 2016 Sep;48(9):1030-4. PMID: 27321543

Nachman F, Vazquez H, Gonzalez A, Andrenacci P et al, Gastroesophageal reflux symptoms in patients with celiac disease and the effects of a gluten-free diet. Clin Gastroenterol Hepatol. 2011 Mar;9(3):214-9. PMID: 20601132

Roland BC, Ciarleglio MM, Clarke JO, Semler JR et al. Low ileocecal valve pressure is significantly associated with small intestinal bacterial overgrowth (SIBO). Dig Dis Sci. 2014 Jun;59(6):1269-77. PMID: 24795035

Fialho A, Fialho A, Schenone A, Thota P et al. Association between small intestinal bacterial overgrowth and deep vein thrombosis. Gastroenterol Rep (Oxf). 2016 Nov;4(4):299-303. PMID: 27044499

Reddymasu SC, McCallum RW. Small intestinal bacterial overgrowth in gastroparesis: are there any predictors? J Clin Gastroenterol. 2010 Jan;44(1):e8-13. PMID: 20027008

Capurso G, Signoretti M, Archibugi L, Stiliano S et al. Systematic review and meta-analysis: Small intestinal bacterial overgrowth in chronic pancreatitis. United European Gastroenterol J. 2016 Oct;4(5):697-705. PMID: 27733912

Fialho A, Fialho A, Schenone A, Thota P et al. Association between small intestinal bacterial overgrowth and deep vein thrombosis. Gastroenterol Rep (Oxf). 2016 Nov;4(4):299-303. PMID: 27044499

Bures J, Cyrany J, Kohoutova D, Förstl M et al. Small intestinal bacterial overgrowth syndrome. World J Gastroenterol. 2010 Jun 28;16(24):2978-90. PMID: 20572300

Lake-Bakaar G, Quandros E, Beidas S, et al. Gastric secretory failure in patients with acquired immunodeficiency syndrome (AIDS). Ann Intern Med 1988; 109:502-4. PMID: 3137856

Rana SV, Bhardwaj SB. Small intestinal bacterial overgrowth. Scand J Gastroenterol. 2008;43(9):1030-7. PMID: 18609165

Small Intestinal Bacterial Overgrowth: Clinical Presentation in Patients with Roux-en-Y Gastric Bypass. Obes Surg. 2021 Feb;31(2):564-569. PMID: 33047289

Mathias JR, Clench MH. Review: pathophysiology of diarrhea caused by bacterial overgrowth of the small intestine. Am J Med Sci. 1985 Jun;289(6):243-8. PMID: 3890541

Naseem Z, Premaratne G, Hendahewa R, "Less is more": Non operative management of short term superior mesenteric artery syndrome. Ann Med Surg (Lond). 2015 Oct 23;4(4):428-30. PMID: 26904194

Kaur A, Pawar NC, Singla S, Mohi JK et al. Superior Mesentric Artery Syndrome in a Patient with Subacute Intestinal Obstruction: A Case Report. J Clin Diagn Res. 2016 Jun;10(6):TD03-5. PMID: 27504378

Liakakos T, Thomakos N, Fine PM, Dervenis C, et al. Peritoneal adhesions: etiology, pathophysiology, and clinical significance. Recent advances in prevention and management. Dig Surg. 2001;18(4):260-73. PMID: 11528133

Vane DW, Shiffler M, Grosfeld JL, Hall P et al, Reduced lower esophageal sphincter (LES) pressure after acute and chronic brain injury. J Pediatr Surg. 1982 Dec;17(6):960-4. PMID: 7161684

Gabbard SL, Lacy BE, Levine GM, Crowell MD. The impact of alcohol consumption and cholecystectomy on small intestinal bacterial overgrowth. Dig Dis Sci. 2014 Mar;59(3):638-44. PMID: 24323179

Lo WK, Chan WW. Proton pump inhibitor use and the risk of small intestinal bacterial overgrowth: a meta-analysis. Clin Gastroenterol Hepatol. 2013 May;11(5):483-90. PMID: 23270866

Kim G, Deepinder F, Morales W, Hwang L et al. Methanobrevibacter smithii is the predominant methanogen in patients with constipation-predominant IBS and methane on breath. Dig Dis Sci. 2012 Dec;57(12):3213-8. PMID: 22573345

Youn YH, Park JS, Jahng JH, Lim HC, et al. Relationships among the lactulose breath test, intestinal gas volume, and gastrointestinal symptoms in patients with irritable bowel syndrome. Dig Dis Sci. 2011 Jul;56(7):2059-66. PMID: 21240630

Kim KM, Kim B-T, Lee D-J, Park S-B et al. Erosive esophagitis may be related to small intestinal bacterial overgrowth. Scand J Gastroenterol. 2012 May;47(5):493-8. PMID: 22416969

Eisenmann A, Amann A, Said M, Datta B et al, Implementation and interpretation of hydrogen breath tests. J Breath Res. 2008 Dec;2(4):046002. PMID: 21386189

Costa MB, Azeredo IL, Marciano RD, Caldeira LM et al. Evaluation of small intestine bacterial overgrowth in patients with functional dyspepsia through H2 breath test. Arq Gastroenterol. 2012 Dec;49(4):279-83. PMID: 23329223

Logan AC, Beaulne TM. The treatment of small intestinal bacterial overgrowth with enteric-coated peppermint oil: a case report. Altern Med Rev. 2002 Oct;7(5):410-7. PMID: 12410625

Chedid V, Dhalla S, Clarke JO, Roland BC et al. Herbal therapy is equivalent to rifaximin for the treatment of small intestinal bacterial overgrowth. Glob Adv Health Med. 2014 May;3(3):16-24. PMID: 24891990

Kwak DS, Jun DW, Seo JG, Chung WS et al. Short-term probiotic therapy alleviates small intestinal bacterial overgrowth, but does not improve intestinal permeability in chronic liver disease. Eur J Gastroenterol Hepatol. 2014 Dec;26(12):1353-9. PMID: 25244414

Stotzer PO, Blomberg L, Conway PL, Henriksson A et al. Probiotic treatment of small intestinal bacterial overgrowth by Lactobacillus fermentum KLD. Scand J Infect Dis. 1996;28(6):615-9. PMID: 9060066

Khalighi AR, Khalighi MR, Behdani R, Jamali J et al. Evaluating the efficacy of probiotic on treatment in patients with small intestinal bacterial overgrowth (SIBO)--a pilot study. Indian J Med Res. 2014 Nov;140(5):604-8. PMID: 25579140

Ong DK, Mitchell SB, Barrett JS, Shepherd SJ et al. Manipulation of dietary short chain carbohydrates alters the pattern of gas production and genesis of symptoms in irritable bowel syndrome. J Gastroenterol Hepatol. 2010 Aug;25(8):1366-73. PMID: 20659225

Pimentel M, Constantino T, Kong Y, Bajwa M et al. A 14-day elemental diet is highly effective in normalizing the lactulose breath test. Dig Dis Sci. 2004 Jan;49(1):73-7. PMID: 14992438

SEVENTEEN

BILE REFLUX: THE NEXT VALVE DOWN CAN REFLUX TOO!

The next valve down can reflux too,
Be careful whatever you do,
If bile's the issue,
To protect your tissue,
The options for treatment are few.

GLOSSARY

acetylcholine—the major neurotransmitter for the vagus nerve and "gut brain"

acetylcholinesterase inhibitor—various natural or synthetic substances which delay the breakdown of acetylcholine and improve parasympathetic nervous system activity

acetyl-L-carnitine—an amino acid that is converted into acetylcholine

bile duct stent—a metal or plastic tube inserted into the common bile duct to improve the flow of bile

bile salts—made in the liver and stored in the gall bladder, these are one of the primary components of bile. Bile salts help with the digestion of fats and fat-soluble vitamins, including A, D, E, and K.

binding or binders— bile acid binders (also called sequestrants) bind to bile acids and prevent their reabsorption in the intestines.

biopsy—a small sample of a body tissue that is examined microscopically to aid diagnosis of diseases

cholecystectomy—surgical removal of the gall bladder

colon—the last part of the digestive tract before the anus—also known as the large intestine.

common bile duct—the tube that carries bile from the liver to the sphincter of Oddi and small intestine

cystic duct—the tube that carries bile from the gall bladder to the common bile duct and small intestine

deoxycholic acid—a secondary bile salt

erosions—loss of mucus membrane surface cells, more shallow than an ulcer

erythema—redness caused by increased blood in tissue

hepatocytes—the cells that make up the majority of the liver's structure and function

HIDA scan—a type of diagnostic imaging that reveals bile flow in channels from the liver to the gall bladder and out into the intestine

5- hydroxytryptophan— an amino acid that is converted into the hormones serotonin and melatonin

lecithin—a component of bile that, along with bile salts, emulsifies fat and water

lithocholic acid—a secondary bile salt

peristalsis—the coordinated muscular wave pattern that moves food, bacteria and waste from mouth to anus

petechiae—pinpoint bright red areas of bleeding into tissues

pyloric valve—a thickened area of muscle at the bottom of the stomach. It controls the flow of food and fluid from the stomach to the duodenum.

reactive gastropathy—changes seen on biopsy when the stomach lining is irritated by various substances over time. These substances include nonsteroidal anti-inflammatory drugs (NSAIDs), alcohol, and bile.

serotonin reuptake inhibitor (SSRI)—a group of antidepressant medicines that raise the serotonin level in the synaptic space between nerve cells.

sphincter of Oddi—the muscular valve that opens to allow bile to flow from bile ducts to the small intestine

sphincterotomy—incision of the sphincter of Oddi to allow a gallstone to pass into the intestine

tauroursodeoxycholic acid—an anti-inflammatory bile salt used as an oral medicine

terminal ileum—the last portion of the small intestine

ursodeoxycholic acid— an anti-inflammatory bile salt used as an oral medicine

KEY QUESTIONS

How does bile reflux complicate GERD and treatment-resistant GERD?

What are the symptoms of bile reflux and how is it diagnosed?

What treatments may help bile reflux?

Digestion is said to be a north to south process—normally, everything moves down from mouth to anus. Bile reflux is the reverse flow of bile. Instead of moving down, it refluxes up through the pyloric valve and into the stomach. Not much is known about what causes this, but it is much more common after surgeries for the stomach and gall bladder as well as for bile duct structures.

NORMAL BILE FLOW AND FUNCTION

Bile is a mixture of cholesterol, **lecithin** and **bile salts** produced in the liver and stored in the gall bladder. When a meal containing fat or protein leaves the stomach, the gall bladder contracts, propelling bile though the **cystic duct**, **common bile duct** and **sphincter of Oddi** into the upper small intestine. One of bile's important functions is to emulsify fat and water. This allows most dietary fat, including essential fatty acids (such as those in fish oil) and the fat-soluble vitamins A, D, E and K to be properly digested so that they can be absorbed into the blood.

After bile is released into the duodenum, it flows through the 18-20 feet of the small intestine to eventually be reabsorbed in the **terminal ileum**. 95% of the bile is absorbed into the blood and therefore only about 5% enters the **colon**. If too much bile enters the large intestine, it acts

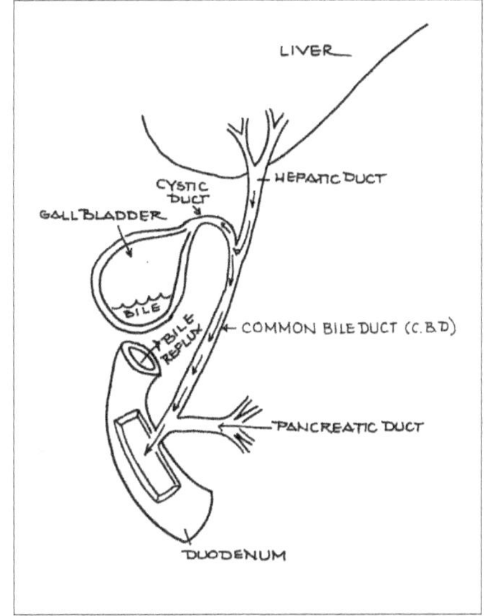

Fig. 17.1. The billary tree.

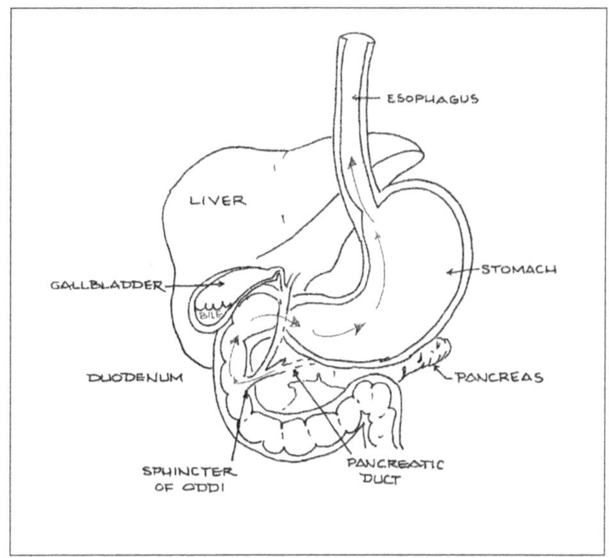

Fig. 17.2. Reflux of bile from duodenum to esophagus.

as an irritant and can cause a form of severe diarrhea called bile acid diarrhea.

BILE GASTRITIS OR ESOPHAGITIS DUE TO BILE REFLUX

The irritant effects of bile, pancreatic and intestinal enzymes in the stomach can cause bile acid gastritis. If these secretions reflux from the stomach into the esophagus, the mix may increase the severity of esophagitis and Barrett's esophagus (Sun D, 2015).

Bile gastritis is diagnosed by upper endoscopy with biopsy. On scope exam there may be **erythema**, greenish bile staining of the gastric mucosa or obvious pooling of bile in the stomach. In addition, there may be visible thickening of the folds of the stomach lining, **erosions**, or signs of small amounts of bleeding into the tissue called **petechiae**. In some cases, bile reflux may be diagnosed on a **HIDA scan** (Eriksson B, 1998).

A **biopsy** of the gastric mucosa will reveal inflammation referred to as **reactive gastropathy** alternately described as chemical gastropathy or reflux gastropathy. When stomach pH is measured in those with extensive bile reflux, the range is between mildly acid and alkaline (5.5-8.0) because that is the pH range to be expected in the small intestine (Othman AAA, 2021).

SYMPTOMS AND EFFECTS OF BILE REFLUX

The symptoms of bile reflux can range from mild to extreme. The most common symptoms I have seen in my patients include low

Bile reduces dietary fat into small droplets so it can be digested by pancreatic lipase.

appetite, nausea, vomiting after meals and burning upper abdominal pain. If the bile refluxes from the stomach into the esophagus or throat, patients may suffer from typical GERD symptoms. It is also likely that they will get little relief from standard acid blocking drug treatments, because bile is very irritating to the mucus lining in the stomach, esophagus, and throat—whether it is mixed with stomach acid or not. In addition, some research shows that chronic bile reflux may increase the damaging effect of stomach acid on the lower esophagus. Barrett's esophagus, the long-term complication of GERD described in the next chapter, may be more severe in those who also have bile reflux. There is evidence from research in rats that even in the absence of gastric acid, exposure of the lower esophagus to secondary bile salts can cause Barrett's esophagus (Sun D, 2015). Up to 68% of those experiencing GERD who have not had gallbladder surgery and do not get relief from standard PPI medication have bile reflux, meaning they have both reflux of stomach secretions and bile (Monaco L, 2009).

When bile refluxes into the stomach, it typically causes nausea, stomach pain and loss of appetite.

If the bile refluxes further up into the esophagus, it causes GERD symptoms, but these are rarely relieved by standard GERD treatments.

GASTRIC SURGERY AND BILE GASTRITIS

Despite the high incidence of bile reflux described above, a factor that increases the chance of having bile gastritis is any gastric surgery that damages the pyloric sphincter. In addition, bile organ procedures, such as **cholecystectomy**, **sphincterotomy**, and **bile duct stent** placement, increase the likelihood of sphincter of Oddi malfunction (Kuran S, 2008).

BILE REFLUX TREATMENTS

Common treatments that I recommend for bile reflux fall into six categories.

- Lowering high intra-abdominal pressure levels that promote reflux

- Improving bile composition

- Protecting the mucosa from bile

- **Binding** bile to remove it

- Strengthening the LES and **pyloric valve** to prevent reflux through either of these valves

- Improving **peristalsis**, the coordinated muscular wave pattern that moves food, bacteria, and waste from mouth to anus

LOWERING INTRA-ABDOMINAL PRESSURE

Although more research is needed, increased abdominal gas raises intra-abdominal pressure (Carry PY, 1994). High pressure restricts the diaphragm's function and promotes upward flow of abdominal contents. Small intestine bacterial overgrowth (SIBO) and intestinal methanogen overgrowth (IMO) increase intra-abdominal pressure. Treatments for SIBO and IMO were discussed in chapter sixteen. Low fermentation diets, herbal antibiotics, rifaximin and related prescription antibiotics or elemental diet can all be used as treatments. In my experience, reducing abdominal gas relieves pressure and reduces reflux.

IMPROVING THE BILE COMPOSITION

Bile is composed of bile salts, lecithin and cholesterol.

In the small intestine, bacteria convert primary bile salts into secondary bile salts.

Reducing the corrosive effects of bile on the stomach and lower esophagus may prevent further irritation. The major components of bile are cholesterol, lecithin, and bile salts—also called bile acids. Primary bile salts are produced in the **hepatocytes** of the liver. Later, when secreted into the small intestine, the bile salts will be converted into secondary bile salts by intestinal bacteria. Secondary bile salts include **deoxycholic acid** and **lithocholic acid**, known to be irritants and even carcinogens. Taking proton pump inhibitors increases bacterial overgrowth in the stomach (Tsuda A, 2015 and Del Piano M, 2014). Just as with small intestine bacteria, gastric bacteria can convert bile that has refluxed into the stomach into irritating secondary bile salts (Sital RR, 2006).

Unique forms of secondary bile salts called **tauroursodeoxycholic acid (TUDCA)** and **ursodeoxycholic acid (ursodiol)** make up only 2% of the total pool of bile salts in the human gall bladder and intestine. Unlike other bile salts that are pro-inflammatory and pro-oxidant, TUDCA and ursodiol have anti-inflammatory and antioxidant effects. It is believed that these benefits are due to ursodiol's ability to increase glutathione, one of the major antioxidant substances in the body (Souza RF, 2016). Taking either of these bile salts as oral medicines may reduce the damaging effects of other secondary bile salts.

As mentioned above, **lecithin** is a normal component of bile. Research shows that it helps protect the cells lining the digestive tract from the irritant effects of bile salts (Narain PK, 1998). It can be supplemented orally to increase lecithin concentrations (Dial EJ, 2008).

PROTECTING THE MUCOSA FROM BILE

In a rodent study, curcumin, a turmeric extract, was more effective than a proton pump inhibitor in preventing esophagitis due the combination of acid and bile. This protective effect is attributed to turmeric's antioxidant and anti-inflammatory properties (Mahattanadul S, 2006).

BINDING BILE TO REMOVE IT FROM THE STOMACH

Cholestyramine is the most effective bile acid binder that has been researched, with more than 90% of bile acids adsorbed at all pH values studied. Sucralfate adsorbs about 50% of bile acids and works best at less acidic pH range. The antacids aluminum hydroxide, magnesium hydroxide, magnesium carbonate or aluminum-magnesium hydroxide antacids, were found to be significantly less effective than cholestyramine. Aluminum hydroxide was the most effective of these mineral antacids, especially at highly acidic pH range (Stahlberg M, 1987).

Other binders are available, but I have not found bile acid research for these that was done in a living gut (Gannasin SP, 2016 and Lund ED, 1984).

STRENGTHENING THE LOWER ESOPHAGEAL SPHINCTER AND PYLORIC VALVE

Acetylcholine is the main parasympathetic neurotransmitter for the enteric nervous system—the unique "second brain" that controls the functions of the sphincters, peristaltic muscular motility, secretion of enzymes, acid, bicarbonate, and absorption of nutrients. The tenth cranial nerve, also called the vagus nerve, connects the brain in the skull with the brain in the gut. Many techniques can be used to tone the vagus nerve such as mindfulness, breath techniques, heart rate variability training (Gerritsen RJS, 2018) as well as exercises for the upper throat. These include therapeutic gargling, humming, singing, and the IQoro device (see https://www.iqoro.com/#). Also helpful are alternate nostril breathing and other types of diaphragmatic breathing. See https://hmmpdx.com/videos for videos on alternate nostril and diaphragmatic breathing techniques.

Huperzine A is an extract of the Chinese herb *Huperzia serrata*. It is best known for its memory enhancing effects. Huperzine A is an **acetylcholinesterase** inhibitor which delays the breakdown of acetylcholine the way a **serotonin reuptake inhibitor** (**SSRI**)

Acetylcholine is the neurotransmitter for the parasympathetic pathways of the vagus nerve.

The vagus nerve connects the brain and gut.

Acetylcholine is essential for the proper functioning of the sphincters in the digestive tract.

delays the breakdown of serotonin. Lecithin, also known as phosphatidylcholine, and other sources of the B vitamin choline, may serve as a precursor to acetylcholine (Wiedeman AM, 2018). More acetylcholine increases the tone of the sphincters and may therefore be helpful in reflux. Thorough chewing (as discussed in chapter eleven) may help vagal parasympathetic tone. A study found that reduced or poor chewing caused significant increases in reflux and disordered swallowing (Pauletti RN, 2022).

IMPROVING PERISTALSIS

The treatments I have discussed above also improve peristalsis, but prokinetics are the most direct treatments to aid muscular contraction of the GI tract. Prokinetics are herbal or prescription substances that promote muscular activity and downward flow of chyme and stool through the gut.

Prokinetics especially suited to the stomach and small intestine

- Low dose erythromycin. This low dose prescription is about a fifth of that used for antibiotic effects.

- Low dose naltrexone. This low dose prescription is about a tenth of that used for treatment of narcotic addiction.

- *Zingiber officinale* (ginger root)

- Motility Activator™—a combination of extracts from ginger root and *Cynara cardunculus* (artichoke).

Prokinetics that may promote stomach, small intestine and large intestine activity

- Prucalopride (brand names Motegrity™ in the USA and Resolor™ in Canada) by prescription

- Iberogast™—an over-the-counter herbal combination prokinetic, anti-spasmodic, and carminative. *Iberis amara* (bitter candytuft) is the main prokinetic herb in the formula.

- MotilPro™—a combination of vitamin B6, ginger root, **acetyl-L-carnitine and 5-hydroxytryptophan**

BILE REFLUX—A COMPLEX CONDITION

Bile reflux is an under-researched and poorly understood medical condition. It is complex and needs to be treated in a highly individualized fashion. It should be distinguished from gastroparesis, biliary dyskinesia, and other types of reflux. There is hope for improvement if one pursues an organized, thorough approach that recognizes and addresses underlying causes.

CITATIONS

Sun D, Wang X, Gai Z, Song X et al. Bile acids but not acidic acids induce Barrett's esophagus. Int J Clin Exp Pathol. 2015 Feb 1;8(2):1384-92. PMID: 25973022

Eriksson B, Emas S, Jacobsson H, Larsson SA et al. Comparison of gastric aspiration and HIDA scintigraphy in detecting fasting duodenogastric bile reflux. Scand J Gastroenterol. 1988 Jun;23(5):607-10. PMID: 3399834

Othman AAA, Dwedar AAZ, ElSadek HM, AbdElAziz HR. Bile reflux gastropathy: Prevalence and risk factors after therapeutic biliary interventions: A retrospective cohort study. Ann Med Surg (Lond). 2021 Dec; 72: 103168. PMID: 34934491

Souza RF, From Reflux Esophagitis to Esophageal Adenocarcinoma. Dig Dis. 2016; 34(5): 483–490. PMID: 27331918

Tack J Koek G, Demedts I, Sifrim D et al. Gastroesophageal reflux disease poorly responsive to single-dose proton pump inhibitors in patients without Barrett's esophagus: acid reflux, bile reflux, or both? Am J Gastroenterol. 2004 Jun;99(6):981-8. PMID: 15180713

Monaco L., Brillantino A., Torelli F., Schettino M., et al. Prevalence of bile reflux in gastroesophageal reflux disease patients not responsive to proton pump inhibitors. World J. Gastroenterol. 2009;15(3):334–338. PMID: 19140233

Kuran S., Parlak E., Aydog G., Kacar S., et al. Bile reflux index after therapeutic biliary procedures. BMC Gastroenterol. 2008;8(1):1–7. PMID: 18267026

Carry PY, Banssillon V. [Intra-abdominal pressure]. Ann Fr Anesth Reanim. 1994;13(3):381-99. PMID: 7992945

Tsuda A, Suda W, Morita H, Takanashi K et al. Influence of Proton-Pump Inhibitors on the Luminal Microbiota in the Gastrointestinal Tract. Clin Transl Gastroenterol. 2015 Jun 11;6(6):e89. PMID: 26065717

Del Piano M, Pagliarulo M, Tari R, Carmagnola et al. Correlation between chronic treatment with proton pump inhibitors and bacterial overgrowth in the stomach: any possible beneficial role for selected lactobacilli? J Clin Gastroenterol. 2014 Nov-Dec;48 Suppl 1:S40-6. PMID: 25291126

Sital RR, Kusters JG, De Rooij FWM, Kuipers EJ et al. Bile acids and Barrett's oesophagus: a sine qua non or coincidence? Scand J Gastroenterol Suppl. . 2006;(243):11-7. PMID: 16782617

Narain PK, DeMaria EJ, Heuman DM. Lecithin protects against plasma membrane disruption by bile salts. J Surg Res. 1998 Aug;78(2):131-6. PMID: 9733630

Dial EJ, Rooijakkers SHM, Darling RL, Romero JJ et al. Role of phosphatidylcholine saturation in preventing bile salt toxicity to gastrointestinal epithelia and membranes. J Gastroenterol Hepatol. 2008 Mar;23(3):430-6. PMID: 17868333

Mahattanadul S, Radenahmad N, Phadoongsombut N, Chuchom T et al. Effects of curcumin on reflux esophagitis in rats. J Nat Med. 2006 Jul;60(3):198-205. PMID: 29435885

Stahlberg M, Jalovaara P, Laitinen S, Mokka R et al. Adsorption of bile acids by sucralfate, antacids, and cholestyramine in vitro. Clin Ther. 1987;9(6):615-21. PMID: 3440273

Gannasin SP, Adzahan NM, Mustafa S, Muhammad K. Techno-functional properties and in vitro bile acid-binding capacities of tamarillo (Solanum betaceum Cav.) hydrocolloids. Food Chem. 2016 Apr 1;196:903-9. PMID: 26593571

Lund ED. Cholesterol binding capacity of fiber from tropical fruits and vegetables. Lipids. 1984 Feb;19(2):85-90. PMID: 6323908

Gerritsen RJS, Band GPH. Breath of Life: The Respiratory Vagal Stimulation Model of Contemplative Activity. Front Hum Neurosci. 2018 Oct 9;12:397. PMID: 30356789

Wiedeman AM, Barr SI, Green TJ, Xu Z et al. Dietary Choline Intake: Current State of Knowledge Across the Life Cycle/ Nutrients. 2018 Oct 16;10(10):1513. PMID: 30332744

Pauletti RN, Callegari-Jacques SM, Fornari L, Iran de Moraes, J. Reduced masticatory function predicts gastroesophageal reflux disease and esophageal dysphagia in patients referred for upper endoscopy: A cross-sectional study. Dig Liver Dis. 2022 Mar;54(3):331-335. PMID: 34645595

EIGHTEEN

COMPLICATIONS OF CHRONIC REFLUX: BARRETT'S ESOPHAGUS

When chronic reflux threatens to harm,
The tissue can't just sit there unarmed.
Instead, it compels
Itself to change cells,
And Barrett's the result of this charm.

GLOSSARY

diagnostic tests - tests intended for those showing symptoms or signs of a disease and in need of a diagnosis.

differentiation of cells - differentiated cells are those that have changed in form and matured from being generalized (such as a stem cell) into being more specific in terms of function.

dysplastic – precancerous cells that may be found in various tissues and are less differentiated than healthy cells

screening tests – tests used to check for early signs of common diseases and are intended for those who have no known symptoms

KEY QUESTIONS

What are the possible complications of chronic GERD?

What are the methods for screening and diagnosing Barrett's?

What are the factors that increase the risk of developing Barrett's?

Which lifestyle factors and natural supplements are protective against Barrett's?

BARRETT'S AND ITS RISKS

The immune system constantly surveys the physical and chemical status of membranes lining all the body's organs. It monitors and responds to irritation or infection with inflammation. Chronic reflux, as discussed in chapter two, may lead to such inflammation. When inflammation is excessive and prolonged, however, the lower esophagus may develop shallow erosions or deeper ulcers. Another response may be Barrett's esophagus (BE, also called "Barrett's"), marked by cellular changes that can increase the risk of progression to cancer.

BE is a change in the cells lining the lower esophagus. The change is a type of metaplasia, an adaptive cellular response. This cellular change is the esophageal lining's attempt to protect itself from long term exposure to stomach contents.

Barrett's esophagus is a type of metaplasia, an adaptive cellular response to the chronic irritation of GERD.

The reason Barrett's is of concern is that a tiny fraction of BE cases may progress to **dysplasia,** a precancerous change, or, even further, to esophageal cancer. Over the past 30 years the incidence of esophageal adenocarcinoma (EAC) has increased more than any other cancer in developed nations. Women have one-sixth the risk compared to men. The good news, however, is that these more severe complications of GERD are quite rare (0.4-0.5% per year) and effective early treatment often prevents dysplasia and cancer (Duits LC, 2019). Unfortunately, less than 10% of patients get screened for this cancer or early changes that can lead to it.

For a more extensive analysis of proton pump inhibitors and Barrett's esophagus go to https://drjournalclub.com/ let's-be-real-about-reflux/

Factors That Increase the Risk of Barrett's

According to Zhou Z et al, (2021), the following factors have been found to increase the risk of developing BE:

- caucasian status
- male sexual status
- abdominal obesity
- type 2 diabetes
- sleeping less than 6 hours/night
- age over 50
- history of smoking

Zhou et al also found that taking PPIs was associated with developing Barrett's. This association is due to the high likelihood that patients with chronic reflux often take PPIs, rather than to a causal relationship.

Men with at least two other risk factors should be screened for Barrett's esophagus, according to the American College of Gastroenterology.

Protections Against Barrett's

A recent meta-analysis based on over 60 international research studies found the following factors <u>protective</u> to varying degrees against developing Barrett's esophagus (Zhou Z, 2021):

- taking aspirin
- taking statin drugs
- increased vitamin C intake
- increased folic acid intake
- increased fiber intake
- eating less meat (less significant)
- sleeping 8 or more hours/night

The researchers reported that the quality of most of the included studies was high and the results significant.

SCREENING FOR AND DIAGNOSING BARRETT'S ESOPHAGUS AND ITS COMPLICATIONS

First, what's the difference between screening and diagnosing? It all depends on whether the patient is symptomatic. Screening tests are intended for those who have no known symptoms, whereas diagnostic tests are intended for those showing symptoms or signs in need of a diagnosis.

Currently the best test for BE is the upper endoscopy (EGD). With the EGD, the lower esophagus is viewed through a scope and biopsies can be taken for microscopic examination. Biopsy is the definitive diagnostic test which proves the presence of Barrett's and checks for possible complications—dysplasia or adenocarcinoma. Areas suspicious for BE usually appear reddened or salmon-colored and velvety compared to the surrounding normal esophageal mucosa which appears pale and glossy. When seen, these areas are measured and listed as short segment (measuring up to 3 centimeters in length) or long segment (greater than 3 centimeters in length). A coordinated study done among multiple research centers in the US and the Netherlands found that patients with short segment have a significantly lower annual rate of progression to cancer of 0.07% compared to 0.25% in patients with long segment (Hamade N, 2019).

Men with at least two of the other risk factors listed above, should have EGD screening for Barrett's, even if they do not have heartburn or other symptoms of GERD. This is especially true for white males over 50 years of age, who are obese and/or are current smokers (An Updated ACG Guideline, April 2022). Family history of Barrett's or esophageal adenocarcinoma are also strong indicators for screening. Because females have a very low risk, this test is only performed to diagnose other esophageal problems, but not to screen for Barrett's.

Biopsy is the diagnostic test, but the pathologists reading the biopsies don't always agree on the diagnosis. Because of this, it is recommended that a second pathologist analyze the biopsy specimens performed on patients suspected of having BE. Always get a second opinion.

A standard feature in endoscopy is called virtual chromoendoscopy which is a blue light used for inspecting the esophagus of patients with Barrett's. It makes it easier to see important early changes in the lining and blood vessels. Some gastroenterologists neglect to use this, but according to the ACG Guidelines for gastroenterologists, "The blue light lets you pick up early mucosal and vascular changes which might represent dysplastic lesions. It's not a question of should. It's a medicolegal slam dunk; you must do it."

NEW TECHNOLOGIES MAY MAKE BARRETT'S TESTING ACCURATE, LESS EXPENSIVE, AND LESS INVASIVE

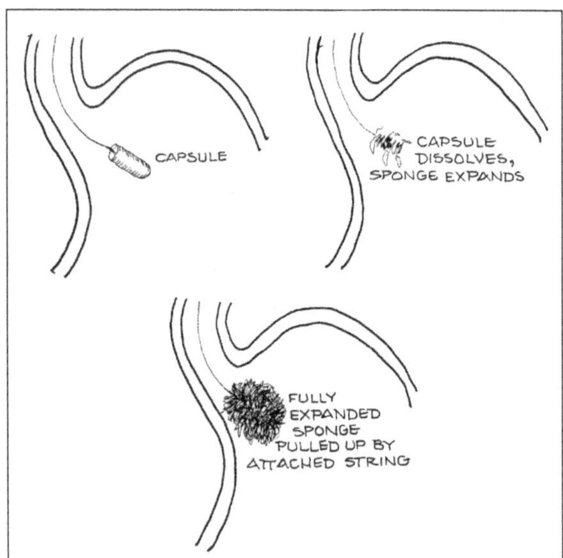

18.1. Cytosponge screening for Barrett's esophagus.

The Cytosponge is already in use in the United Kingdom, and the EsoCheck and EsoCap are in development for use in the United States to screen for BE and esophageal cancer. EsoGuard is a more sophisticated device already available in the United States (www.esoguard.com). All of these tests are designed for in-office use and don't require sedation. Similar to a PAP smear that collects cells from the uterine cervix, these tests brush cells from body tissues to allow DNA analysis or microscopic exam. A thin plastic tube is used in Esoguard. The others use a small sponge which is packed into a capsule and attached to a string. As the capsule is swallowed, the string unwinds down into the stomach. The capsule dissolves rapidly, the sponge opens and is then pulled up through the esophagus. During this process the sponge gathers cells and DNA which can be analyzed by pathologists for the presence of Barrett's, dysplasia and gene mutations that increase the risk of progression from BE to adenocarcinoma (Duits LC, 2019).

HOW CAN THE PROGRESSION OF BARRETT'S TO ESOPHAGEAL CANCER BE PREVENTED?

Since the chronic inflammation driving Barrett's metaplasia is often caused by GERD, it has long been assumed that neutralizing the pH of the stomach will protect from dysplasia and adenocarcinoma. Curiously, the research on this topic has been complex. Please go to https://drjournalclub.com/let's-be-real-about-reflux/ for an expert analysis of this data.

A 2017 meta-analysis did not find evidence for this idea, stating:

> In summary, no definitive protective effects against the development of esophageal adenocarcinoma and/or high-grade dysplasia were seen for patients with Barrett's with long-term PPI usage. Until and unless results of future studies can confirm such an association, PPI usage should be restricted to symptom control according to current guidelines. These findings indicate that for an unselected group of patients with BE, chemoprevention by use of PPIs to reduce progression should not be considered directly as routine care. (Hu C, 2017).

A newer study of proton pump inhibitor use showed a significant reduction in the progression of Barrett's to high grade dysplasia or adenocarcinoma (Chen Y, 2021). Based on these findings, the American College of Gastroenterology came out with a new practice guideline saying, "We suggest at least once a day PPI therapy in patients with BE without allergy or other contraindication for PPI use" (ACG guideline, April 2022). Unfortunately, they rated the quality of this evidence as "very low" and the strength of the recommendation as "conditional". If you find this confusing, you are not alone.

It is my hope that PPIs *do* protect people from complications, rather than increasing risks. In my practice, additional options for protection include treating the cause of reflux whenever possible and using diet, nutritional supplements, and botanical medicines.

MY KEY OBJECTIVES:

- <u>control or correct reflux by treating the cause, whenever possible</u>

- prevent Barrett's from developing in the esophagus of those with chronic reflux

- prevent progression to dysplasia in areas already affected by Barrett's metaplasia

- increase **differentiation of cells**. A differentiated cell has changed in form and matured from being generalized (such as a stem cell) into being more specific in terms of function. **Dysplastic** esophageal cells are less differentiated than healthy esophageal cells.

- promote healing of esophagitis

RECOMMENDATIONS INCLUDE:

Fresh vegetables and fruits

Increasing consumption of fresh produce is associated with a lower risk for developing BE in men and women (Thompson OM, 2009). Use of berry extracts are common for this purpose to increase the consumption of important antioxidant compounds such as flavonoids and beta carotene. Beta carotene may prevent the progression to Barrett's esophagus with dysplasia (Ibiebele TI, 2013).

Adequate dietary B vitamin intake

A study of over 900 subjects included almost equal number of controls as well as those with EAC, BE, and erosive esophagitis. EAC risk decreased with increasing folic acid intake. Similar findings were seen for BE and erosive esophagitis. Vitamin B2 (riboflavin) intake was inversely associated with erosive esophagitis (Sharp L et al, 2013).

Vitamins C and E

Research proves that for people under age 65, vitamin C has significant protective effects against developing Barrett's esophagus and esophageal adenocarcinoma. This benefit was seen for those with both higher dietary vitamin C intakes as well as higher blood levels of vitamin C. In this younger age group, there were also significant protective effects against developing esophageal adenocarcinoma from higher vitamin E intake (Kang JH et al, 2018).

Treat SIBO if present

Treating SIBO is important to reduce secondary bile salts such as deoxycholic acid. Increasing numbers of bacteria in the upper small intestine lead to excessive production of secondary bile salts which form free radicals. Also referred to as reactive oxygen species, free radicals are involved in DNA damage to the cells that become Barrett's cells (Mudyanadzo TA, 2018 and Champion G, 1994)

Turmeric

In a rodent study, curcumin, an extract of turmeric root, has been shown to prevent the esophageal mucosal damage induced by reflux esophagitis. Curcumin was more effective than a proton pump inhibitor in preventing esophagitis due to bile-acid reflux. This protective effect is attributed to turmeric's antioxidant and anti-inflammatory properties (Mahattanadul S, 2006).

Green tea catechins including epigallocatechin gallate (EGCG)

Studies have demonstrated a protective effect for green tea consumption against developing and dying from a variety of human cancers. These include breast, esophagus, stomach, and blood cancers. At doses of 400-600 mg per day, EGCG accumulates in the esophageal mucosa (Koe AK, 2015). It prevents the growth of cells at high risk of developing into esophageal adenocarcinoma (Song S, 2009).

Melatonin and Tryptophan

One possible reason why sleeping less than 6 hours per night is a risk factor for Barrett's may be sleep's relationship to melatonin. Whether supplementation of melatonin or tryptophan, its precursor, can protect BE from developing into EAC requires more research. Considering the safety of melatonin supplementation (or getting 8 hours of sleep per night) I see no reason to avoid its use prior to this being proven significant (Majka J, 2018).

CITATIONS

Hur C, Miller M, Kong CY, Dowling EC et al. Trends in esophageal adenocarcinoma incidence and mortality. Cancer. 2013 Mar 15;119(6):1149-58. PMID: 23303625

Duits LC, Lao-Sirieix P, Wolf QA, O'Donovan M et al. A biomarker panel predicts progression of Barrett's esophagus to esophageal adenocarcinoma. Dis Esophagus, 2019 Jan; 32(1): doy102. PMID 30496496

Zhao Z. Yin Z, Zhang C. Lifestyle interventions can reduce the risk of Barrett's esophagus: a systematic review and meta analysis of 62 studies involving 250,157 participants. Cancer Med. 2021 Aug; 10(15): 5297–5320. PMID: 34128354

Hamade N, Vennelaganti S, Parasa S, Vennalaganti P et al. Lower Annual Rate of Progression of Short-Segment vs Long-Segment Barrett's Esophagus to Esophageal Adenocarcinoma. Clin Gastroenterol Hepatol. 2019 Apr;17(5):864-868. PMID: 30012433

Middleton DRS, Mmbaga BT, O'Donovan M, Abedi-Ardenkani B et al. Minimally invasive esophageal sponge cytology sampling is feasible in a Tanzanian community setting. Int J Cancer. 2021 Mar 1;148(5):1208-1218. PMID: 33128785

Hu C et al. Proton Pump Inhibitors Do Not Reduce the Risk of Esophageal Adenocarcinoma in Patients with Barrett's Esophagus: A Systematic Review and Meta-Analysis. PLoS One. 2017 Jan 10;12(1):e0169691. PMID: 28072858

Chen Y, Sun C, Wu Y, Chen X, et al. Do proton pump inhibitors prevent Barrett's esophagus progression to high-grade dysplasia and esophageal adenocarcinoma? An updated meta-analysis. _J Cancer Res Clin Oncol. 2021 Sep;147(9):2681-2691. PMID: 33575855

Shaheen NJ, Falk GW, Iyer PG, Souza RF et al. Diagnosis and Management of Barrett's Esophagus: An Updated ACG Guideline, Official journal of the American College of Gastroenterology | ACG117(4):559-587, April 2022. PMID: 35354777

Thompson, OM et al. Vegetable and fruit intakes and risk of Barrett's esophagus in men and women. Am J Clin Nutr. 2009 Mar;89(3):890-6. PMID: 19144726

Ibiebele TI, Hughes MC, Nagle CM, Bain CJ et al. Dietary antioxidants and risk of Barrett's esophagus and adenocarcinoma of the esophagus in an Australian population. Int J Cancer. 2013 Jul;133(1):214-24. PMID: 23292980

Sharp L, Carsin A-E, Cantwell MM, Anderson LA et al. Intakes of dietary folate and other B vitamins are associated with risks of esophageal adenocarcinoma, Barrett's esophagus, and reflux esophagitis. J Nutr. 2013 Dec;143(12):1966-73. PMID: 24132576

Kang JH, Luben R, Alexandre L, Hart AR et al. Dietary antioxidant intake and the risk of developing Barrett's oesophagus and oesophageal adenocarcinoma. Br J Cancer. 2018 Jun 12; 118(12): 1658–1661. PMID: 29780162

Koe AK, Schnoll-Sussman F, Bresalier RX, Abrams JA et al. Phase Ib Randomized, Double-Blinded, Placebo-Controlled, Dose Escalation Study of Polyphenon E in Patients with Barrett's Esophagus. Cancer Prev Res (Phila). 2015 Dec; 8(12): 1131–1137. PMID: 26471236

Mudyanadzo TA. Barrett's Esophagus: A Molecular Overview. Cureus. 2018 Oct 19;10(10):e3468.

PMID: 30585284

Champion G, Richter JE, Vaezi MF, Sigh S et al. Duodenogastroesophageal reflux: relationship to pH and importance in Barrett's esophagus. Gastroenterology. 1994 Sep;107(3):747-54. PMID: 8076761

Mahattanadul S, Radenahmad N, Phadoongsombut N, Chuchom T et al. Effects of curcumin on reflux esophagitis in rats. J Nat Med. 2006 Jul;60(3):198-205. PMID: 29435885

Song S, Krishnan K, Kiu K, Bresalier RS, et al. Polyphenon E inhibits the growth of human Barrett's and aerodigestive adenocarcinoma cells by suppressing cyclin D1 expression, Clin Cancer Res. 2009 Jan 15;15(2):622-31. PMID: 19147768

Majka J et al. Melatonin in Prevention of the Sequence from Reflux Esophagitis to Barrett's Esophagus and Esophageal Adenocarcinoma: Experimental and Clinical Perspectives. Int J Mol Sci 2018 Jul; 19(7): 2033. PMID: 30011784

NINETEEN

GER AND GERD IN INFANTS AND CHILDREN

Kids can have reflux too.
Infants often spit up their food,
But when weight gain is flagging,
With choking or gagging,
GERD treatments should then be pursued.

GLOSSARY

gastroesophageal reflux (GER)—normal minimal amounts of reflux

regurgitate—the passage of refluxed contents into the pharynx or mouth also called spitting-up (in infants)

KEY QUESTIONS

How common is GERD in infants and children?

What are the symptoms of GERD in infants?

Is regurgitation abnormal in infants?

How is the treatment of GERD in infants and children different from the treatment in adults?

Does the nursing mother's diet or the formula for bottle-fed infants influence GERD?

INFANTS AND GER

Reflux from the stomach into the esophagus can occur at any age. As discussed previously, reflux, or **gastroesophageal reflux (GER)** is a normal phenomenon, but if it causes distress, pain or damage to the esophagus, pharynx, or upper airway tissues, it is GERD.

A systematic review of research published over the last 23 years revealed that about a third-to-a-half of all healthy infants **regurgitate** at least once a day. This peaks at four months of age and 90% of them are over this tendency by their first birthday (Poddar U, 2019 and Chabra S, 2020). Adolescents and adults also have a more minor form of benign GER, with an average of three minimal reflux events after each meal. These normal reflux events are usually imperceptible and cleared by secondary peristalsis.

Less than 2% of infants suffer from GERD. By adolescence, the incidence is about the same as adult GERD (20%).

Testing for **GERD**

Testing for GERD in infants and children is rarely done unless there are red flags such as:

- failure to grow or gain weight

- choking, gagging, or coughing during nursing

- movements or postures indicating the baby is in pain

- blood in the milk that is spit up

It is important to realize that GERD can cause symptoms and disease in other body areas besides the upper digestive tract, such as earaches, sinus problems, coughing, refusing feeding, fussiness, and sleep disruption (Berger WE, 2007 and Hassall E, 2005).

Treatments

There is little support to suggest that the use of proton pump inhibitors improves the symptoms of GERD in infants. PPIs *are not* effective in healing the child's esophageal lining (Poddar U, 2019). The older H2 receptor antagonists, such as famotidine, are considered more appropriate if prescription treatment is chosen. Older children, as well as adolescents, may receive either PPIs or H2 receptor antagonists.

Non-drug Treatments

Most infants, children, and adolescents with reflux respond to non-drug treatments. In breastfeeding infants, the nursing mother may experiment with a trial of avoiding certain foods. Commonly reactive foods such cow's milk or eggs may improve the nursing child's reflux. As a first approach for formula-fed infants, using smaller or more frequent feedings may decrease reflux episodes (Rosen R, 2018). Hypoallergenic hydrolyzed protein or elemental amino acid formulas may reduce reflux in infants allergic to cow's milk (Lightdale JR, 2013).

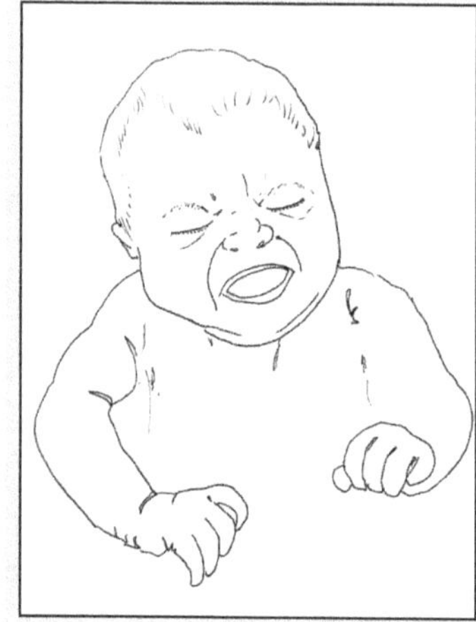

Fig.19.1. Babies don't fuss without a reason.

Less than 2% of infants suffer from GERD. By adolescence, the incidence is about the same as adult GERD (20%).

While awake, the baby's position after nursing or bottle feeding may be an important factor. Lying face down or on the left side may be helpful (Rosen R, 2014), but the consensus of the North American and European pediatric gastroenterology groups did not find adequate support to make this recommendation. Please remember that sleeping infants (under age one year) should always be in the face up position to decrease the risk of sudden infant death syndrome.

LIFESTYLE FACTORS

For older children and adolescents with GERD, consider my mnemonic for the possible significant lifestyle factors—Reduce CARBS—relieve reflux (see chapter eight). Most children should not be placed on a low carbohydrate diet, but the type of carbohydrates consumed may need to be changed for therapeutic effect. Work with a nutritionist or nutrition trained physician before changing a child's diet.

CITATIONS

Poddar U. Gastroesophageal reflux disease (GERD) in children. Paediatr Int Child Health. 2019 Feb;39(1):7-12. PMID: 30080479

Chabra S, Peeples ES. Assessment and Management of Gastroesophageal Reflux in The Newborn. Pediatr Ann. 2020 Feb 1;49(2):e77-e81. PMID: 32045486

Berger WE, Schonfeld JE. Nonallergic rhinitis in children. Curr Allergy Asthma Rep. 2007 May;7(2):112-6. PMID: 17437681

Hassall E. Decisions in diagnosing and managing chronic gastroesophageal reflux disease in children. J Pediatr. 2005 Mar;146(3 Suppl):S3-12. PMID: 15758900

Rosen R, Vanderplas Y, Singendonk M, Cabana M et al. Pediatric Gastroesophageal Reflux Clinical Practice Guidelines: Joint Recommendations of the NASPGHAN and ESPGHAN. J Pediatr Gastroenterol Nutr. 2018 Mar;66(3):516-554. PMID: 29470322

Lightdale JR, Gremse DA. Gastroesophageal reflux: management guidance for the pediatrician. Pediatrics. 2013;131(5):e1684–e1695. PMID: 23629618

Rosen R. Gastroesophageal reflux in infants: more than just a pHenomenon. JAMA Pediatr. 2014;168(1):83–89. PMID: 24276411

TWENTY

REFLUX AND SEX

Females feel GERD with more intensity,
While the damage to males has more immensity.
Estrogen protects,
From esophageal defects,
'Til menopause removes estrogen's density.

KEY QUESTIONS

How does the patient's sex affect the symptoms and risk for progression in GERD?

How do risk factors for GERD vary between the sexes?

Why might women have less risk of the advanced complications of GERD?

SEX-BASED RISK FACTORS, SYMPTOMS, AND RISK OF ESOPHAGITIS IN GERD

A review of 96 research papers on sex and reflux found that risk factors for reflux esophagitis in women include age over 70 years, obesity, elevated blood triglycerides, central obesity (waist circumference greater than 35.0 inches*), current smoking status, and hiatal hernia. Women—both before and after menopause—experience more heartburn, regurgitation, and extra-esophageal symptoms such as cough and hoarseness. They also have a higher incidence of NERD. After age 70, women have increased incidence of erosive esophagitis—prior to 70, it is significantly less common in women than in men (Kim SY, 2016 and Kim SY, 2019).

On the other hand, risk factors for reflux esophagitis in men include overweight or obese status, hypertension, elevated blood triglycerides, central obesity (waist circumference greater than 40 inches*), current or past tobacco smoking, excessive alcohol consumption, and hiatal hernia. For men, advancing age does not appear to be a significant risk factor. Males are more likely than females to develop Barrett's, advance to dysplasia, and esophageal adenocarcinoma.

---

* The Korean Society for the Study of Obesity recommends the cut-off of 33.4 inches for Korean women and 35.4 inches for Korean men (Koh JH, 2010).

A British endoscopy study found that both men and women have a 7% increase in development of Barrett's esophagus over a lifetime. For men, this increase started at age 20, but in women it was delayed until age 40. The 20-year age lag caused a two-fold male predominance for Barrett's (van Blankenstein M, 2005). Large Dutch and Irish studies found similar results (van Soest EM, 2005 and Coleman HG, 2011). Delayed development of Barrett's for women gives men up to a 9-fold increased risk for developing esophageal cancer. It is believed that this protective effect is due to estrogen levels in premenopausal women.

ESTROGEN AND **GERD**

Research suggests that estrogen may protect the esophageal mucosa. The mechanism appears to be improved esophageal tight junctions (Orlando LA, 2009). Recall from chapter three that virtually everyone with GERD has dilated intercellular spaces ("leaky esophagus"). The intercellular space is narrowest in NERD and widest in Barrett's (Alvaro-Villegas JC, 2010). A study found that giving estrogen to male rabbits reduced the risk of dilated intercellular spaces in response to various esophageal irritants. Lower levels of estrogen in men may be a factor that causes a higher prevalence of reflux esophagitis and Barrett's (Honda J, 2016). Female estrogen levels prior to menopause may explain the decreased prevalence of reflux esophagitis in women until after age 50. Estrogen has been shown to reduce growth and increase destruction of abnormal cells in Barrett's esophagus and esophageal cancer (Sukocheva OA, 2013). In addition, a Swedish population-based study of over 200,000 women showed that hormone replacement therapy for women has a protective effect against esophageal adenocarcinoma. Hormone treatment also reduced the odds of developing stomach cancer. Both estrogen-only hormone replacement and combination estrogen and synthetic progesterone were significantly protective in all age groups. (Brusselaers N, 2017).

Lower levels of estrogen may explain the increased risk of reflux esophagitis and Barrett's in men.

Hormone replacement therapy in women may protect against esophageal adenocarcinoma.

CITATIONS

Kim YS, Kim N, Kim GW. Sex and Gender Differences in Gastroesophageal Reflux Disease. J Neurogastroenterol Motil. 2016 Oct 30;22(4):575-588. PMID: 27703114

Kim SY, Jung HK, Lim J, Kim TO. Gender Specific Differences in Prevalence and Risk Factors for Gastro-Esophageal Reflux Disease. J Korean Med Sci. 2019 Jun 2;34(21):e158. PMID: 31144481

van Blankenstein M, Looman CW, Johnston BJ, et al. Age and sex distribution of the prevalence of Barrett's esophagus found in a primary referral endoscopy center. Am J Gastroenterol 2005;100:568–76. PMID: 15743353

van Soest EM, Siersema PD, Dieleman JP, et al. Age and Sex Distribution of the Incidence of Barrett's Esophagus Found in a Dutch Primary Care Population. Am J Gastroenterol 2005;100:2599–600. PMID: 16279923

Coleman HG, Bhat S, Murray LJ, et al. Increasing incidence of Barrett's oesophagus: a population-based study. Eur J Epidemiol. 2011 Sep;26(9):739-45. PMID: 21671079

Koh JH, Koh SB, Lee MY, Jung PM et al. Optimal Waist Circumference Cutoff Values for Metabolic Syndrome Diagnostic Criteria in a Korean Rural Population. J Korean Med Sci. 2010 May; 25(5): 734–737. PMID: 20436710

Alvaro-Villegas JC et al. Dilated intercellular spaces in subtypes of gastroesophagic reflux disease. Rev Esp Enferm Dig. 2010 May;102(5):302-7. PMID: 20524757

Honda J, Iijima K, Asanuma K, et al. Estrogen enhances esophageal barrier function by potentiating occludin expression. Dig Dis Sci. 2016;61:1028–1038. PMID: 26660903

Sukocheva OA, Wee C, Ansar A, Hussey DJ et al. Effect of estrogen on growth and apoptosis in esophageal adenocarcinoma cells. Dis Esophagus 2013 Aug;26(6):628-35. PMID: 23163347

Brusselaers N et al. Menopausal hormone therapy and the risk of esophageal and gastric cancer. Int J Cancer. 2017 Apr 1;140(7):1693-1699.   PMID: 28006838

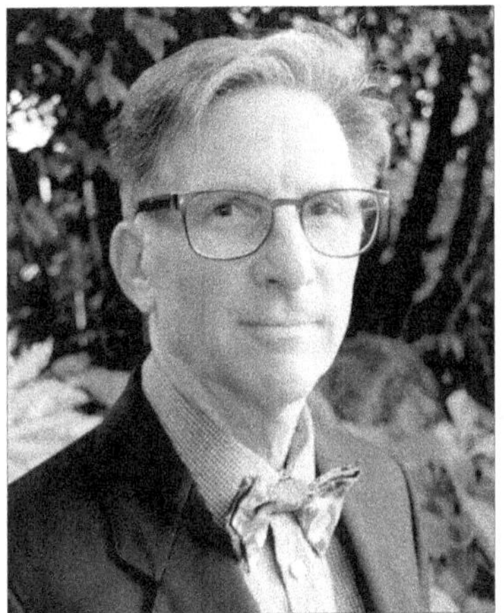

Steven Sandberg-Lewis, ND, DHANP, received his doctorate from the National College of Naturopathic Medicine, now the National University of Natural Medicine (NUNM) in Portland, OR, USA in 1978. He has been in continuous private practice for 45 years and is in his third decade as a professor of gastroenterology at NUNM.

He is frequently interviewed and lectures nationally and internationally at seminars and webinars. In addition to *Let's Be Real About Reflux*, he is the author of the textbook, *Functional Gastroenterology: Assessing and Addressing the Causes of Functional Gastrointestinal Disorders* (2017 second edition).

Sandberg-Lewis is one of the founders of the GastroANP, the Gastroenterology Association of Naturopathic Physicians.

In addition to working with patients in Oregon and California where he is licensed to practice Naturopathic Medicine, he conducts educational consultations with physicians and people suffering from digestive disorders throughout the other 48 states and internationally.

His websites include:
www.hmmpdx.com
www.functionalgastroenterology.com

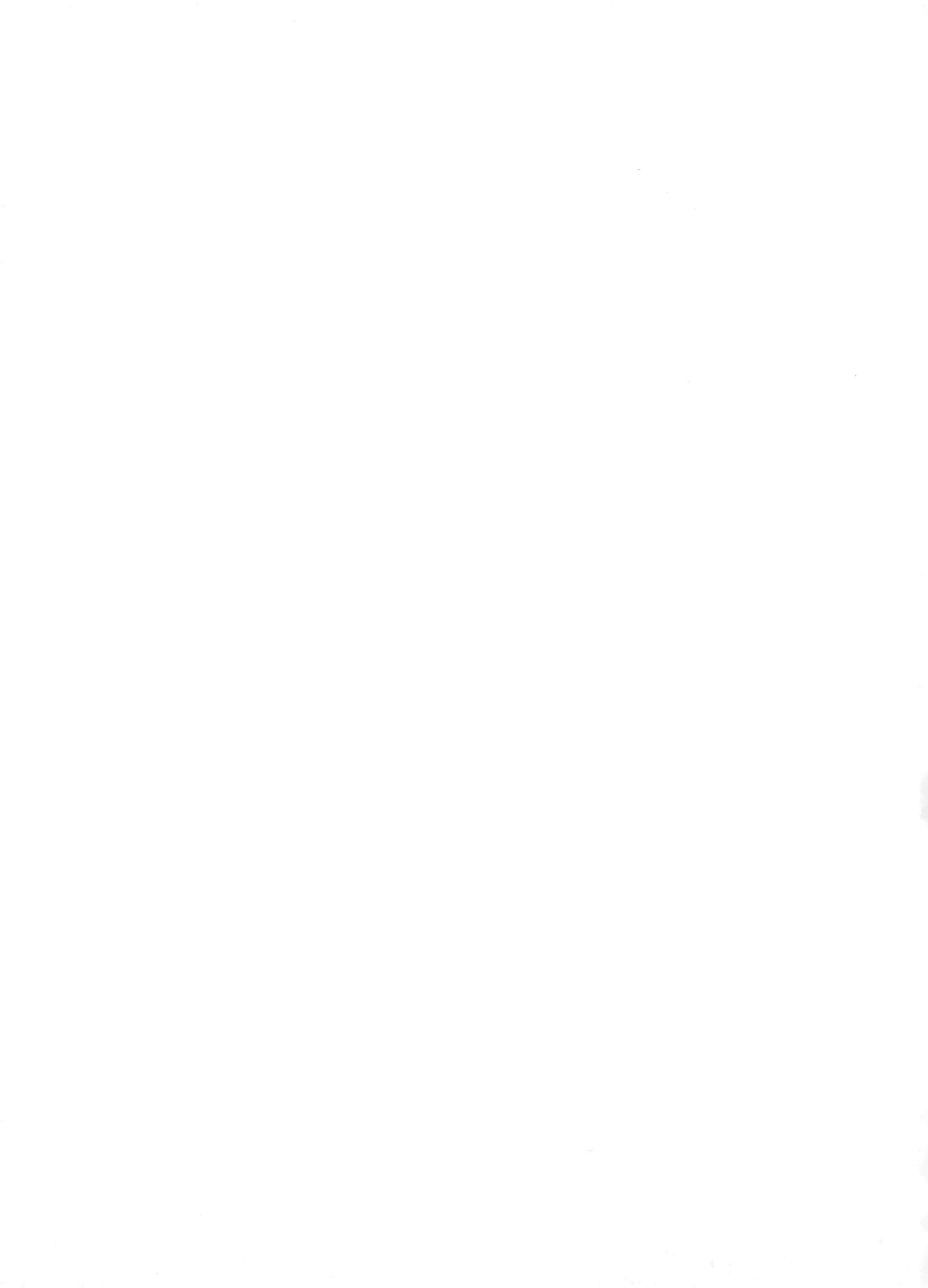